Praise for
The Activity Kit for Babies and Toddlers at Risk

"I had the tremendous fortune of previewing this book and being coached by the authors when my daughter was diagnosed with autism spectrum disorder at 14 months old. We actually had fun incorporating the creative activities into our daily lives. Along with therapy, these techniques undoubtedly contributed to my daughter's amazing progress. Reading this book is like having these four leading consultants guiding you in your home every step of the way!"
—Stephanie S., parent

"Fantastic! The book provides key information about typical developmental milestones from birth through toddlerhood, and is chock full of clever games and activities to make learning fun."
—Wendy Stone, PhD,
Director, READi Lab (Research in Early Autism Detection and Intervention), University of Washington

"I will recommend this book to all the parents I work with. It is just what you need if you are worried about your infant's or toddler's development. The chapters are bursting with easy-to-implement games and activities, embedded in daily routines, that could help any child."
—Sally Ozonoff, PhD, coauthor of *A Parent's Guide to High-Functioning Autism Spectrum Disorder, Second Edition*

"A marvelous, unique resource that fills an important need. This book is filled with practical and helpful advice and activities that parents can readily use when developmental delays are suspected. It enables you to take active steps to facilitate your child's development."
—Fred R. Volkmar, MD, coauthor of *A Practical Guide to Autism*

"This clearly written, extremely user-friendly book will be invaluable to parents. It contains a plethora of ingenious ideas that you can incorporate into your everyday routines to enhance and expand your young child's learning."
—Katarzyna Chawarska, PhD,
Yale Child Study Center, Yale University School of Medicine

THE ACTIVITY KIT
FOR BABIES AND TODDLERS AT RISK

The Activity Kit
for Babies
and Toddlers
at Risk

How to Use Everyday Routines to Build
Social and Communication Skills

Deborah Fein, PhD
Molly Helt, PhD
Lynn Brennan, EdD, BCBA-D
Marianne Barton, PhD

THE GUILFORD PRESS
New York   London

Library of Congress Cataloging-in-Publication Data

Fein, Deborah.
    The activity kit for babies and toddlers at risk : how to use everyday routines to build social and communication skills / Deborah Fein, Molly Helt, Lynn Brennan, and Marianne Barton.
        pages   cm
    Includes bibliographical references and index.
    ISBN 978-1-4625-2091-6 (pbk. : alk. paper)
    1. Developmentally disabled children—Behavior modification.   2. Parents of developmentally disabled children.   3. Developmental disabilities—Treatment.   I. Title.
    RJ506.D47F45 2016
    649'.151—dc23
                                                                        2015025239

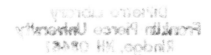

To Elizabeth and Emily (D. F.),

Matty and Jack (M. H.),

Ben (L. B.),

and Megan and Kelsey (M. B.),

*who have taught us so much about parenting
and who give us so much joy*

Contents

PART II
Games and Activities
for Toddlers at Risk

PART III
Games and Activities
for Babies at Risk

PART IV
More Tips and Tools

Acknowledgments

We wish to acknowledge first and foremost the thousands of parents of children with autism and other neurodevelopmental conditions whom we have gotten to know over the years. Their understanding of their children—their patience, devotion, and wisdom—has taught us an incredible amount. We also want to thank all the early intervention therapists and other clinicians whose dedication and skill have been such an inspiration. Thank you as well to the wonderfully skilled editors and other staff at The Guilford Press, who were an absolute joy to work with on this book, especially Kitty Moore, Chris Benton, Carolyn Graham, and Lucy Baker.

D. F.: I want to thank Harriet Levin. In the almost 30 years we've worked together, I have watched your clinical talent with awe and learned so much from you about young children. I also want to thank my husband, Joe, who is endlessly patient and wise, and my daughters, Liz and Emily, who are the light of my life. I'm also very grateful to be in such a supportive department (Psychology) and university (University of Connecticut—go Huskies!!). Last, but not least, I want to express my thanks to my brilliant and generous coauthors and colleagues: to Molly, whose amazing creativity and experience as a professional and as a parent gave rise to most of the activities in the book; to Lynn, who is the best behavior analyst I have ever worked with; and to Marianne, whose gentle wisdom and understanding of attachment are unparalleled.

M. H.: I want to thank my sons, Matty and Jack; our respective journeys together inspired many of the activities in this book. I love you to infinity and beyond. I would also like to thank my husband and best friend, Marc, who always encourages and always believes in the happy ending around the corner. I am grateful to my parents for showing me what a joyful experience parenting is under any circumstances, and for making it possible for me to pursue this work that is so meaningful to me. Last, but not least, I thank my brilliant and dedicated coauthors, who have helped countless families and children thus far in their careers and inspired me to want to do the same. I particularly thank Deborah Fein, who has been my mentor, role model, and friend for the past decade and who continues to inspire me with her wisdom, generosity, and grace.

L. B.: I want to thank all of my coauthors and especially Deborah Fein, who is as kind, generous, and supportive as she is intelligent, knowledgeable, and principled. Deb, working so closely with you for the past 6 years has added a great deal to my life both professionally and personally. I also want to thank my husband, Kevin, and son, Ben, whose love and friendship are everything to me.

M. B.: I want to thank the many graduate students whose energy and thoughtful questions have made this work great fun and kept us all thinking carefully. I also want to thank my husband, David, who has been my steadfast partner in all things, and my daughters, Megan and Kelsey, who are the great joy of my life. And I thank all of my coauthors, especially Deborah Fein, who has been a brilliant, wise, and generous collaborator on so many projects over the years.

Authors' Note

Everything included in this book applies both to male and female children and to male and female parents, as well as to other caregivers. We have used "Mommy" when illustrating what to say to your baby or toddler more often than any other term, just for simplicity's sake. Obviously, you will substitute "Daddy," "Grandma," or whatever other name you use with the child. We have also used "Baby" in activity names and when illustrating how to speak to your child, and you should naturally substitute your child's name. Finally, we alternate between masculine and feminine personal pronouns throughout the book.

Introduction

IS THIS BOOK FOR YOU?

"My 2-year-old is not saying any words and not understanding very much of what we say to him. While we're waiting for a language evaluation, is there anything we can do?"

"Our 18-month-old is showing signs of autism. He's not looking at us and not speaking or pointing. We know these are signs of an autism spectrum disorder but can't get him evaluated for another 6 months. What can we do in the meantime?"

"The psychologist who diagnosed my 2-year-old with autism spectrum disorder recommended intensive therapy, but we can only get 1 hour a week. What can we do to make up for some of this time?"

"We have a 6-year-old who has autism and want to give our 6-month-old baby the best possible start. Is there anything we can do to enrich his environment?"

"We adopted our baby at 9 months, and she doesn't seem to smile as much or make as much eye contact as other babies. Is there anything we can do to enrich her environment?"

This book is for parents in all of these and similar situations. Over many years, we've heard from or talked to thousands of parents who want to know how to help a very young child who is at risk for autism spectrum disorder (ASD) or another developmental delay. Maybe the child has received a preliminary diagnosis or your pediatrician has expressed concern about your child's social or language development.

1

Perhaps you have an infant who is at risk for an ASD (the baby was born at a very low birth weight or prematurely, has tuberous sclerosis, or has an older sibling with ASD) and you want to ensure you are providing a stimulating environment to give your baby the best possible start. You could be in the common and understandably frustrating situation of either having to wait months for a diagnostic evaluation, or being on a waiting list for early intervention, or even being told to "wait and see." You don't want to waste any time; you want to know what you can do at home to boost your child's development and minimize delays starting right now, whether your child is a few months or a few years old.

An ASD (see the box below) is a developmental disorder characterized by deficits in social communication and social interaction. Of all developmental disorders it is probably the best defined and described, and so the clearest body of research on successful intervention exists for children who have at least some characteristics of ASD. But ASD shares many features with other developmental conditions, including global developmental delay and developmental language disorder. For example, children with developmental language disorder also struggle to tell adults what they want or need, and they may have a hard time understanding language without gestures or pointing. Children with global developmental delays often benefit from having extra practice at learning, thinking, and language skills. Children who are adopted after the age of 6 months may benefit from extra activities that encourage attachment and social connection. The games and activities we describe in this book should be helpful and fun for children at risk for many kinds of developmental concerns. In fact, we believe these activities would even be helpful for children with typical development!

NEW TERMINOLOGY

In the new diagnostic system (DSM-5), *autism spectrum disorder* refers to all the conditions related to autism—including autistic disorder, pervasive developmental disorder not otherwise specified (PDD-NOS), Asperger syndrome, atypical autism—that were used in older systems. In this book, we use "autism spectrum disorder" or "ASD" interchangeably with "autism" to refer to the group of autism-related conditions. We use this terminology to make clear that we are referring to the broader category of disorders, which are very hard to differentiate in young children, and because the activities we describe are likely to be helpful to children across the autism spectrum.

The age we're targeting is birth to 3 years, although you should be able to continue to use the ideas in this book for older children as well.

If the child is receiving professional intervention, consult with your therapist about which activities would be best to help your child generalize what he is being taught in therapy; that is, applying what he is learning to different situations.

The choice of which activities to try is really up to you—see if your child is ready for each activity and which ones he enjoys.

WHAT DO WE MEAN BY "AT RISK"?

There are two kinds of children we might consider at risk for a developmental delay or disorder.

First is the child who is showing some concerning behaviors or delays. For example, an 18-month-old child who is not showing a lot of attention to your speech or understanding what you say to her, or who has no words of her own, may be experiencing a language delay of a few months. If your 12-month-old is not pointing or making eye contact, he may have a social delay. Spending a lot of time staring at things in an unusual way and tuning you out is of concern in a 2-year-old. Mild delays of a few months are often temporary, and the child will catch up, especially if the delay is an isolated one. If, for example, your 18-month-old is walking, handling objects, interacting with adults socially, and understanding what you say to him at the level expected for his age, but is not yet saying words, that is more likely to be a temporary issue than if he has delays in more than one of these areas.

If your child is showing some delays or concerning behaviors, he may already have been given a diagnosis, such as ASD, developmental language disorder, or global developmental delay (a delay that affects multiple areas of development). But many pediatricians and specialists do not like to give such a diagnosis until the child is about 3 years old, even if the delays are already pretty clear. In that case, we might call the child "at risk for" autism or another developmental disorder. *So when we talk about the "at-risk" child, we are including the child with observable delays or concerning behaviors, whether or not he has received a diagnosis and whether or not the delays or behaviors are mild, moderate, or severe.*

The second kind of child who might be called "at risk" is not showing any obvious delays or concerning behaviors, but you have other reasons to think she might be at risk for a developmental delay. These reasons might include:

- An older sibling with a developmental disorder such as autism.
- Significant prematurity or low birth weight.
- A difficult pregnancy or delivery that your doctor has told you carries some risk to the child.
- A diagnosis of a genetic or neurological condition that may be associated with developmental delays.
- A medical condition associated with increased autism risk (such as tuberous sclerosis).
- For an adopted child, lack of good developmental stimulation in the early months or an unknown early history.

If you know your child carries some risk, you may not want to wait to see if these delays show up, but get started on providing whatever enrichment you can in the first few years. It does not matter what medical condition may have caused these kinds of delays; the ideas in this book should help your child learn new skills no matter what condition caused the delay.

In this book, we're concerned mostly with delays in social and language functioning. We're not going to deal with fine motor (handling objects) or gross motor (moving his body) issues because these are highly specialized areas that require professional guidance and intervention. So the conditions that the child may be at risk for that we are concerned with in this book generally include autism and related conditions, developmental language disorder, and global developmental delays. In Chapter 1, we describe in more detail what developmental delays look like at different points in the first few years of life. Some children who are at risk for autism or other developmental delays also have difficulties with sensory or motor functioning; this would include children who are visually and/or hearing impaired and children who have severe motor disabilities or delays. These children need very specialized help, and although the same principles of promoting attachment and behavioral teaching will certainly apply to them, some of the activities or goals we describe (following an adult's point to a distant object, making eye contact with the adult, listening to the adult's language) may not apply to these children. Others may apply but will require specialized teaching methods. If you have such a child, please consult your pediatrician and early intervention provider for developmental stimulation activities that will help him.

WHAT SHOULD YOU DO IF YOU'RE CONCERNED ABOUT YOUR CHILD'S DEVELOPMENT?

Don't wait.

First, if you have concerns about any aspect of your child's development or behavior, make an appointment with your child's pediatrician or pediatric provider to discuss these concerns. You can ask the doctor to screen the child for an ASD (once he is 16 months old) or for other developmental delays (at any age). You can ask for a referral to your statewide early intervention program, where your child can be evaluated; if delays are found, he may qualify for early intervention services. See what your doctor says. The doctor may be able to reassure you that what you're concerned about is age appropriate. If you're not convinced, ask for additional screening and a referral to early intervention or to a specialist such as a developmental-behavioral pediatrician or child psychologist. Trust your instincts as a parent (you can best describe your child's behavior), get input from others who know your child (family members, day care providers, etc.), and rely on the expertise of your child's doctor. As a team, you can best meet your child's needs. If your child does get an autism diagnosis, you should be able to qualify for early intervention services in your state; if at all possible, get a Board Certified Behavior Analyst, one who has experience and expertise with young children, to supervise the child's program. In the Resources section at the back of the book, you will find contact information for the Behavior Analyst Certification Board, which can help you find such a person.

Second, consider using the developmental stimulation activities in this book. It's certainly true that early intervention professionals have the knowledge and experience to design the best programs for your child, and you should take advantage of whatever professional help you can get, both in direct service to your child and in giving you advice about working with your child at home. But the number of hours such professionals are able to provide may be quite limited. At the very least, using the activities in this book can supplement whatever professional help is available to you right now and into the coming months and years.

Why should you add these kinds of activities to your day? There is recent research on autism (that may apply to other children as well) showing that their attention to the faces and voices of familiar people, like parents, may be much better than their attention to strangers. Similarly, their ability to understand the feelings and emotional communication of familiar people may be better than their understanding of strangers. For example, in one recent study, children with autism watching cartoons were not affected by listening to strangers laugh, but when their own mother was laughing with them, their laughter increased. This difference between attention to faces and voices of strangers and attention to familiar adults is especially pronounced in children with social–emotional delays or difficulties. *This makes you the most important person in the life of your child with social delays, such as a child at risk for autism. You are your child's first and most important teacher.*

You may be able to get his attention and promote social learning in a way that a professional who sees him once or twice a week cannot. Even if it's hard to get and keep your child's attention and you feel very frustrated or helpless from time to time, be assured that you are a key person in his life and you have the power to help him make important strides. *Importantly, the fact that we are promoting interacting with your child in a particular way does not mean you have been doing anything wrong up until this point.* Most children develop typically regardless of their environment. However, children with social and emotional delays often need *extra practice* with language and social skills, and they often need this practice in a way that makes the language and social signals they are receiving extra clear to them.

Another reason to use the activities in this book is that they can be a lot of fun—for your child and for you—and they won't take much time out of your busy day, because all the activities are designed for use within your daily routines of caring for and playing with your child. From the moment your child wakes up to the time she goes to bed, you have many opportunities to build language, social skills, imitation, and pretend play. This book contains games to play while you dress your child, rhymes and songs to use during mealtimes and chores, ways to enrich development and learning during play and errands, and more. We've tried to make the instructions simple, brief, and straightforward so the activities are easy to learn and remember for use throughout the day. We know they can be helpful for many children, because we've spent thousands of hours applying them in clinical practice, and they are based on reliable scientific research. And you have more than 100 activities to choose from, so the ones you repeat are the ones your child enjoys and engages in. We hope you'll use this "toy box" full of games and activities for a long time to come.

HOW IS THIS BOOK ORGANIZED?

In Part I, we explain the basis of the activities we've designed for the young children at risk. These facts and principles will be very useful as you move through the day with your baby or toddler, helping you choose the best activities, tune in to what your child likes, and determine what's making a difference over time. Chapter 1 describes developmental milestones from birth to age 3 so you can get a better idea of where your child might stand and what targets for learning you might want to focus on. (Ideally, you'll already have the advice of a professional on this as well, but it helps to become informed, and learning these details can enhance your understanding of what you're seeing in your own child.) In Chapter 2, you'll read about the two main ideas behind early intervention, ideas that will be important for you to understand and then keep in mind as you read the rest of the book: the emotional attachment between parent and child and the basic principles of behavioral intervention. In Chapter 3, we offer some general principles and guidelines for stimulating your child's development at home, ideas that you can use to get and keep your child's attention and to begin to teach him some important skills. In Chapter 4, we describe the most important things that you want to help your child learn as early as possible, things like how to imitate other people and how to communicate with simple language and gestures.

In Part II, each chapter is devoted to a specific daily routine that most families do daily or weekly, like waking up and going to sleep, laundry, cooking, playing and cleanup, dressing, and mealtimes. In each chapter, we describe some games and activities that you can do during these times and list the specific skill or skills being targeted.

Part III is devoted to really young children, those from birth to 1 year of age, or for those children whose delays are significant and may be functioning at the level of a much younger child. Most children under 1 year will not be diagnosed with any developmental condition, and you may be concerned only because you have another child with a developmental delay like ASD or general developmental delay, or because you had a difficult pregnancy or delivery, or because your child was born prematurely. But you would still like to enrich the child's environment as much as possible and give your infant the best start you can. These chapters describe activities you can do with a child in the first year of life, including how to adapt some of the toddler activities in Part II for babies. If your child is under age 1 now, you can start with the activities in Part III and then move on to those in Part II as the child grows.

Part IV gives you additional practical tools. First, you'll find a chapter filled with specific words, phrases, signs, and gestures that are appropriate for children under 3 and that you can pick from when working on language and communication. The next chapter suggests communication skills to teach, as well as other strategies, that may help prevent problem behavior like tantrums. At the back of the book you'll find an Appendix that lists all the activities within each daily routine, for both toddlers and babies, keyed to the book page where you'll find the instructions. You might want to photocopy these lists (and even laminate them) to leave in the areas where these routines take place as handy reminders of what you can try with your child. You can also download and print them from *www.guilford.com/fein-forms*. A Resources list—books, organizations, and websites that offer additional helpful information and sources of help—is also at the back of the book.

We hope the activities in this book will offer new strategies for playing with and teaching your child. We believe the interactions that result from these activities will enrich your relationship and build your child's social and communication skills. Most important, we hope you and your child will find new ways to enjoy these early years together.

PART I

HELPING BABIES AND TODDLERS LEARN AND DEVELOP

CHAPTER 1

What Is a Developmental Delay and How Can Games in Routine Activities Help?

When parents become concerned that their children may not be developing as expected, one of their first questions is "Exactly what is a developmental delay?" The best person to answer that question is your child's pediatrician or a specialist like a developmental/behavioral pediatrician or a child psychologist, but here are some general guidelines for some of the major areas of development, especially social–emotional functioning, language, and thinking, up to the age of 3 years. *Please note:* These are very general guidelines. Not every child with typical development will be able to do every single one of these things at the "correct" time. There are also exceptions; for example, children who are adopted internationally during their first year, and did not have the benefit of hearing English for the first 6–12 months of life, are often delayed in their communicative milestones until the third year, when they frequently catch up with their peers. If your child seems to be missing a number of these milestones, do consult with your child's doctor.

3-MONTH-OLDS

By the time a child is 3 months old, she should be able to do the following:

- Coo and perhaps produce a variety of vowel sounds.
- Visually fixate on an object and track it when it moves.
- Lift her head up when she is on her tummy.

- Smile to show pleasure.
- More often than not, stop crying and be able to be soothed when a caregiver attends to her needs.

6-MONTH-OLDS

By the time a child is 6 months old, he should be

- showing a wider range of facial expressions and vocalizations, including laughter.
- able to anticipate some of your actions—that when you bring your hands close to him, you are about to tickle him; when you bring a spoonful of food close to him, you are about to feed him; when you go to the refrigerator, you are about to get him a bottle, etc.
- reaching out his arms when he wants you to pick him up.
- beginning to imitate some of your facial movements (such as sticking out his tongue).
- beginning to take solid food.
- beginning to have a somewhat predictable sleep schedule.
- sitting (or close to sitting) independently.
- most important, paying more and more attention to people by looking at their faces and watching what they do.

9-MONTH-OLDS

By the time a child is 9 months old, she should

- be interested in following the source of her mother's attention (Where is she looking? Where is she pointing?).
- check her mother's face in response to uncertain situations (How does Mommy feel about this stranger?).
- have some meaningful gestures (waving bye-bye, clapping hands) and be able to make some movements associated with songs like "The Itsy Bitsy Spider" or "If You're Happy and You Know It."
- show a clear preference for her caregivers over strangers and be beginning to show you affection by "kissing" (may be more like face sucking) and nuzzling you.
- have a beginning sense of object permanence (knowing that things still exist when they go out of sight) and be interested in games such as "peekaboo."
- be able to reach for the object she prefers from two objects (two shirts, two books, two pieces of food) you hold up.

- have a *beginning* understanding of sharing and turn taking (for example, offering you a bite of her food).
- have the ability to shift her attention back and forth between you and something else (such as a toy you are playing with together).
- be able to recognize the meaning of some words even if she is not yet able to speak.
- be able to show you, by looking at you and either moving her body or vocalizing (though not typically with words), when she wants you to continue an activity.
- smile in response to her parents' smiles, at least some of the time.

1-YEAR-OLDS

By the time of a child's first birthday, most babies demonstrate the following in social and communication skills:

- They know their family members.
- They react differently to people they know well as compared to strangers.
- They like to be hugged by familiar adults or siblings.
- They seek out familiar adults or siblings for comfort if they are hurt or scared.
- Between the ages of about 1 and 2, many children do not want to be separated from their parents; they may cry and fuss when left with an unfamiliar person and cry when they see the parent leave.
- Your child should be looking you in the eye many times each day. Of course, the child may avoid looking at you if he's feeling shy, or teasing you, if he doesn't want to do what you're asking him to do, or if he's very busy with something else, but with familiar people when he's interacting comfortably, there should be a lot of eye contact.
- They enjoy playing back-and-forth games like peekaboo.
- They should understand that when an adult holds out her empty hand, palm facing upward, it means she wants the child to give her something. They may not necessarily do what you want—but they understand what you mean.
- They should enjoy imitating the faces that you make, like a happy, sad, or surprised face, or imitating simple movements or sounds. Most babies aren't very successful at imitating older children or adults, but they think it's fun to try.
- Children by about 1 year old should try to see where you're pointing, even though they may not be very good at it. They should look at an object that you point to if it isn't too far away. They should also look in the direction that you are looking in, especially if you seem very interested in what you are looking at.
- Most babies are starting to point to things they want, although pointing can appear as late as 15 months. They also should be starting to point to things they want to show you.

- When they are interested in something, they should hold it up to show you and bring it over to you to share their interest.
- If they're not sure whether a new sound or object or person is scary, they may look at a parent's face to see how the parent feels about it.
- When you smile at your baby, he should smile back at you most of the time.
- Your baby should also show definite emotions, like happiness, fear, and sadness, and he should be affectionate to family members; 1-year-olds show this affection by hugging, cuddling, or kissing.
- They are interested in their surroundings and pay a lot of attention to both people and objects in their environment.
- Other people should be very important to them, and not just objects. They are also starting to notice how other people feel, so they know when you're happy with them and when you're not.
- When you laugh or show obvious happiness, the baby will at least sometimes respond with smiling or laughing too. They like adults to laugh, and if you laugh at something they do, they might do it again to see you laugh again. They also find it funny when you do something unexpected to amuse them, and they like to have these things repeated. Babies should be happy at least some of the time, with big smiles to show you how joyful they are.
- By the time they are 1 year old, babies should recognize their names. They won't always respond to their name, especially if they're busy with something else, but they know their name, and sometimes they look at you when you call their name.
- They pay attention to people speaking. Most babies can also follow a few simple instructions; for example, if the baby is holding a ball and you hold out your arms and say "Throw the ball" or "Give it to me," or "No!" she should understand you. Of course, she may not want to do what you say or be able to, but you can tell that she understands. Most babies of a year old will understand a few instructions (like "Put it down," "Give it to me," "Throw it," or "Put it on top" with a few different objects—that is, a 1-year-old baby will usually know the difference between "Give me the ball" and "Give me the spoon").
- One-year-olds will understand your tone of voice; that is, they will understand from your voice when you're happy and when you're angry, and they may understand when you're asking a question or expressing surprise.
- The baby who's just past his first birthday may be saying a few words. If not, he should be making a lot of babbling sounds that sound like language (like "ba ba ba").
- Some babies don't say any words until 15 months, and typically the first recognizable words appear between 12 and 18 months. They may not sound much like an adult producing the word, but you can tell that "baba" means "bottle" or "iss iss" means "Elizabeth."

In the development of thinking and attention, you should start to see the following by the age of a year:

- The baby should be very interested in the environment around her. She should notice sounds, like a telephone ringing, at least some of the time. She should be interested in exploring her environment and like to crawl or walk around and see new things. But she likes to look around from time to time and make sure a familiar adult is still around to take care of her. Some children are very bold and like to explore a new environment very actively, while others are more cautious and like to stay close to the familiar adult and only explore in a careful way after getting used to a new place.
- One-year-olds know that if something goes out of their sight, it still exists. So, if they drop something from a chair, they will look for it, for at least a few seconds. If you hide a toy your 1-year-old is playing with under a cloth, he will lift up the cloth to find it. If he drops it off of his high chair or out of his stroller accidentally, he will want it back.
- Many children are not yet doing any pretending at this age, but you might see the beginning of pretend or make-believe play, like holding a toy phone to the ear as if talking or holding an empty cup to the mouth as if drinking.

18-MONTH-OLDS

At this age, the child should have all the skills we talked about for 1-year-olds, and the child should be doing them better and more often, including skills like pointing, looking at your face and your eyes, listening to language, saying a few words, and imitating you. If your child loses skills he or she previously had at any point, it is cause for immediate concern and you should take the child to a specialist to be evaluated. Eighteen-month-olds should

- be pointing pretty often, both to show you what they want and to show you interesting things because they want to share their interest and enjoyment with you. When they point to something, they will often look back at you to make sure you're looking at the right thing.
- enjoy it when adults pay attention to them and watch what they're doing.
- be noticing how adults feel (if they haven't already been doing so). They like adults to be happy and may get upset if the adult, especially a parent or caregiver, is sad or angry or scared.
- be really sure about what they want. They are starting to really assert themselves and may be hard to distract from what they want.
- like to try to help adults do things, even if they cannot really help, like helping you clean or make something in the kitchen.

- be interested in other children, and sometimes like to play *near* other children, although they don't know yet how to really play *with* other children. (An 18-month-old is usually not too happy about sharing his things with other children!)
- be able to imitate simple actions, like clapping hands, or putting his hands on his head, when an adult does it, as well as actions with objects, such as banging on a drum.
- be interested in language and paying attention to adults when the adults talk to them, at least some of the time, even if they cannot always understand what the adults are saying.
- understand a variety of words, phrases, and instructions. They should understand some words for body parts, like "Where's your head?" or clothing items, like "hat," or people, like "Mama," food items, like "cookie" or "juice," simple actions, like clapping, simple adjectives, like "silly" or "big," and highly emotional words such as "yay!" and "uh-oh!"
- be using simple gestures like blowing a kiss or waving bye-bye.
- be saying at least a few words that you can understand. Usually children of this age use their words to ask for the things they want, like "cookie!" or "up!" or "again!" or "more," or they may use their words to show you something interesting; for example, the child might point at a firetruck and say "look!" or try to say "firetruck!" They usually have a name or a word for a parent or caregiver and sometimes call the adult using that word.
- often be able to understand if they are given a choice of two things and reach for the one they want or point to it.
- often be starting to really get the idea of pretend or make-believe, so they may find it fun to pretend some very simple things, like to drink out of an empty cup or hug or feed a stuffed animal or doll.
- be interested in learning new skills and feel proud of themselves when they can do something.
- understand, if they have experience with mirrors, that they are looking at themselves in the mirror.

2-YEAR-OLDS

Between the second and third birthday, you should see all the skills we've talked about for 1-year-olds and 18-month-olds continuing to develop, like eye contact, pointing, imitating, understanding language and speaking, pretending, being interested in other people and how they feel. Remember that if at any time you feel your child is no longer able to do some of the skills previously acquired, it's time to speak with a doctor.

Two-year-olds should also

- be interested in developing more skills, like putting a piece of clothing on or taking it off or feeding themselves.

- be trying to imitate adults doing more complicated things like brushing their hair or wiping a table.

- be getting better at pretend, so they may pretend to do things like feed a baby doll or stuffed animal and pretend to put it to bed or talk on the telephone or pretend to be an animal.

- like learning new skills and showing adults what they have learned.

- interact very actively with adults, saying things to them, looking at their faces, pointing and showing things to the adults, wanting to see what the adults are doing and paying attention to, and playing with them.

- be interested in other children and like to watch them and sometimes to play next to them, but their ability to play together with another child is limited except for physical play like chasing or wrestling.

- be more self-centered than cooperative in their play with another child, wanting the other child's toys and protecting their own toys and finding it difficult to share, especially things they really like.

- understand more language now, so if you say, "Where's the cup?" or "Where's the cat?" they should be able to point to the real thing or a picture of it.

- know several parts of their body (for example, they should point to or touch the right part if you say, "Where's your ear? Where are your eyes? Where's your nose? Where's your mouth? Where's your tummy? Where's your head? Where's your hair? Where are your feet?").

- follow simple directions like "Bring me the key" or "Put the bowl on the table" without needing gestures (for example, a younger child might need you to hold out your hand and point to the key, while the 2-year-old can understand your directions without that). Of course, they won't always cooperate! But if they're paying attention and being cooperative with you, they can do simple things that you ask them to do.

- be starting to speak more, so children at this age should be combining some words into phrases or sentences (for example, they can say "more juice" or "big hat" or "go store" or "Mommy cup").

- start, when 2½ or close to 3, saying longer phrases or even sentences. They can name pictures in a book, like some animals or common household objects. They will be able to refer to themselves as "I" or "me" or by using their name, like they might say "I want juice" or "Me hungry" or "Susie hungry."

- demonstrate a strong sense of what is theirs (or what they wish were theirs!). So you will often hear 2-year-olds saying "mine" or "my cookie" or "my puzzle" very assertively. It may make them difficult to handle sometimes, but it's quite natural.

- be very determined to get what they want and to do things their own way, and if they don't want to do something or don't want someone else playing with their toys, they will let you know. You will probably hear "No!" very often from a 2-year-old.
- understand the idea of making a choice and be able to make choices more consistently and quickly and may say what they want as well as point.
- start to understand the idea of sequence or order, so they can take a small set of things, like three doughnut shapes, and put them in order of size on a peg or take three balls and put them in order from smallest to biggest.
- be able to play with something for a few minutes before losing interest and moving on to something else, although their attention span is still very short.
- be very interested in learning to do things for themselves, like trying to put socks on or pull them off, or trying to put on a pair of pants or shoes. Since they usually have difficulty doing these things by themselves, they may get very frustrated and angry.
- pretend to be an adult, so they may come into the room trying to walk while wearing your shoes or an article of your clothing.

3-YEAR-OLDS

By the age of 3, children become more sociable and develop more advanced communication and language skills. They should

- continue to have good eye contact and joint attention with adults.
- look to parents to see if parents are happy with what they're doing since they want to please them.
- want to play near other children and may be actively playing or talking with them, although at times they may need help to play nicely; for example, they may try to take the other child's toys away without asking or hit another child.
- be starting to understand the idea of taking turns with another child or an adult, although it may be hard for them to wait their turn.
- engage in longer and more complicated pretend play, so they may be able to act out a whole scene, like put a baby doll in a crib, give it a bottle, cover it with a blanket, and say "night-night."
- be able to understand some words that mean a relationship between two things, like understanding the difference between "I'm going *to* the store" and "I'm coming back *from* the store," putting the ball "*on* the table" and putting it "*under* the table."
- be saying many different kinds of things, including putting words together into longer phrases or sentences that are three, four, or five words long.

- be asking some questions, like "Where's Daddy?" or "What's that?"
- be answering those kinds of questions, too, as well as questions like "Are you hungry?" or "What's your name?"
- be making simple comments about things around them that are not just to get their needs met, saying things like "There's Daddy!" or "There's a dog!"
- know some words for objects and animals, but also for actions (like sleep, run, eat, jump).
- be able to tell a boy from a girl and know the words for each.
- be using "ing" on words, like "I'm playing," "I'm singing," instead of just saying "play" or "sing," and they should be putting an "s" on the end of words, like "Mommy's cup" or "two apples."
- have some words for feelings, like "happy," "sad," "scared," and "mad" or "angry."
- be starting to understand what objects are for, so if you say, "What is a fork for?" or "What do we do with a fork?" they can say "eat" or "eating," or if you ask, "What is a bed for?" they will say "sleeping."
- be able to point to something "red" or "yellow" although they may not be able to say these words accurately yet.
- know something about animals, like the sounds made by a cat or a dog, or that cows and horses live on farms, and birds fly and fish swim.
- be starting to understand that certain things go together, so if you give them a bunch of red and yellow pictures mixed together, they can make a pile of red pictures and a pile of yellow pictures or put pictures of animals in one pile and pictures of people in another pile or pictures of birds in one pile and dogs in another pile.
- be able to put on some simple pieces of clothing and take them off although they may get things backward.
- be able to make marks on paper and may be able to draw some simple shapes like circles.

USING THE ACTIVITIES IN THIS BOOK TO BOOST DEVELOPMENT

If you're worried about whether your child's development is delayed based on your observations of your child and the descriptions above, please do see your pediatrician as recommended in the Introduction. Meanwhile, you can start using any of the games and activities in this book with your child. They are designed to stimulate development in the abilities listed in this chapter.

"How Successful Will These Games and Activities Be at Enhancing My Child's Development?"

A lot of clinical experience and research evidence suggests that these activities are likely to stimulate development, but beyond that we can't say exactly how effective they will be for each individual child. There are several reasons we can't.

First, every child is different and has different potential. This may sound like something you've heard so many times that it's meaningless; nevertheless, it's true. Some children will be limited in how quickly they can learn. Others will look delayed in their first few years and then, especially with intensive professional intervention, will speed up and may even catch up completely with other children their age. Furthermore, a professional assessment at an early age may be able to tell you how delayed your child is (or isn't) in different areas at that moment (like thinking, movement, understanding language, producing language, interacting with people). However, unless your child has a specific diagnosable genetic or neurological condition, the assessment will *not* be able to tell you what your child's response to intervention will be, and even with a specific medical diagnosis, there will be a lot of uncertainty. Receiving intensive, high-quality intervention for a couple of years may make it easier to forecast accurately how quickly your child's development will proceed. But when he's still very young (3 or younger) or has not received intensive intervention, forecasting is usually not possible.

Second, in addition to differences among individual children, there are differences among developmental disorders. Children with some disorders tend to have better development than others. Some developmental disorders, like autism, have a huge range of outcomes, with some children facing severe challenges all of their life and others having different kinds and degrees of successful outcomes in social life, school, and adulthood. With other kinds of developmental delays, children who understand language at an age-appropriate level but have trouble producing words tend to catch up more easily than children whose understanding of language is also delayed. Other disorders, such as those involving global developmental delays, will show slower progress. We believe that any child who is experiencing early difficulty with attachment, attention, or language learning should benefit *to some degree* from providing these enriched teaching opportunities; however, the specific gains we can expect from any individual child will vary greatly and depend on his or her underlying biology. Conditions that might cause difficulty with attachment, attention, or language would include children with biological disorders as well as children with environmental deprivation such as those adopted from an orphanage with poor conditions. It is usually not possible to predict a child's developmental potential, and it is never possible without a comprehensive developmental assessment and diagnosis.

Third, the games and activities we describe in this book are based on our collective clinical experience and on a large body of research literature on what helps children learn skills and be securely attached to parents. Nevertheless, a definitive research trial of these games and activities, as a package, and as carried out by parents, to see how effective they are with different types of children, has not been done. We hope to do that study, but in the meantime, we want to offer parents the activities that our clinical experience suggests are likely to stimulate development. And in Chapter 3 you'll find some principles to follow that will increase their effectiveness. **If we were concerned about the development of our own children or grandchildren, these are the things we would do.**

"Could These Games and Activities Be Harmful to My Child?"

We have designed these games and activities to be very similar to games you would do with any children in the course of playing with them, teaching them, and loving them. They are based not only on long-understood behavioral learning methods but also on the natural bond between parent and child, as explained in Chapter 2. This means not only that the activities are likely to have a greater positive effect when done with you than with a stranger but also that, because all children desire connection with their parents, your child is likely to enjoy them. The only way we can imagine them doing harm is if your anxiety about your child's development leads you to communicate that anxiety to the child, to pressure the child into doing things that he cannot yet do, or to get upset with the child when he does not or cannot respond the way you would like. (In fact, it is not uncommon for a parent of a child whose milestones are delayed to experience anxiety or even depression over these delays. If you find yourself in this situation, we strongly recommend seeking the support of a parent group or a professional therapist. You will have the most to offer your child if you are receiving the support you need!) **As long as you keep these activities fun, communicate your enthusiasm and your love, be patient, and keep in mind that a toddler's attention span and effort are limited, they should only be beneficial.**

"How Can I Combine the Ideas in This Book with Professional Intervention?"

As we mentioned earlier, we've been in touch with countless parents who are eager to start helping their child develop communication and social interaction and who don't yet have intensive early intervention, for any number of reasons. If you're lucky enough to have skilled early intervention providers, by all means get their opinion about the games and activities we suggest in this book. If they have other activities to suggest, instead of or in addition to those in this book, we encourage you to give them a try.

There is limited research into just how many hours of intervention are needed for children with general developmental disorders to make the best progress, but the research on ASD is clear: intensive intervention has a generally better outcome than limited intervention, and by "intensive" we mean 20 or more hours a week. We suspect that the more time a child is engaged with people and with his surroundings the better, and that children with ASD may have particular difficulty making use of "down time." For example, when given a toy car and a racetrack to play with, a typically developing child may drive the car all around the race track making car noises, while the child with ASD may become fixated on repetitively rolling the car back and forth in one place, just watching the wheels of the car spin, which has limited developmental benefits, and may even be harmful to the child. Therefore, even if your child is receiving 20 or more hours per week of professional intervention these activities may help you keep him joyfully and purposefully engaged and learning throughout other parts of his day, such as bathtime, feeding, and during errands.

If getting professional intervention for that 20 hours or more is not possible (and this is true for many parents in many U.S. states and regions), you can help make up for that shortfall with the games and activities we describe or by using activities your early intervention provider suggests. You can also help work toward the goals defined by your early intervention provider by choosing activities that are most beneficial in those areas. Chapter 4 describes typical targets of learning, and in Part II we identify the specific skills and concepts targeted by each activity. We've given you many choices of activities within each daily routine not to encourage you to learn and use them all but to absorb the models and the general idea of how to work teaching opportunities into your daily routines. Then you can take the things that are being worked on in your child's professional intervention program and further modify the games and activities to fit those skills.

"How Will I Know If the Extra Stimulation Is Helping?"

You might notice that your child's attention to you is increasing, that she is interested in interacting with you, playing games with you, and listening to you speak. She may also anticipate what you'll do more often and be interested in sharing her enjoyment with you by showing you things, looking into your eyes, and smiling at you. She may be showing more clear emotions, like appropriate smiling, laughing, and crying in response to specific events. Over time, she may seem to understand more of what you say to her. If your child is participating in early intervention, you can ask her therapists what areas of development they are seeing progress in and which they are not. If your child has gotten a formal developmental evaluation, you could ask to have this repeated after 6 months or so to gauge her progress as measured by an expert who can give you more objective feedback.

CHAPTER 2

Keystones

ATTACHMENT AND BEHAVIORAL TEACHING

In this chapter we're going to explain two extremely important ideas: *attachment* and *behavioral teaching*. Then we'll explain how they can go together and how behavioral teaching can be used to increase attachment in young children at risk for a social–emotional disorder such as ASD.

Behavioral teaching/learning (as embodied in applied behavior analysis, or ABA) and stimulating emotional attachment through social interaction form the basis of early intervention. They work together in the most effective interventions. Behavioral approaches can stimulate attachment, and strengthening the child's emotional connection to his caregivers makes a child more responsive to teaching.

ATTACHMENT

Relationships with primary caregivers, often referred to as attachment relationships, are very important to a child's development and especially to the ability to enjoy rich interpersonal interactions. While we know that children at risk for ASD or other developmental disorders can form attachments to their caregivers, they sometimes don't seem to use these attachments to engage in back-and-forth social interactions in the same way as other children do.

Attachment is defined as a strong and affectionate tie that people of all ages feel toward special people in their lives. John Bowlby, an English psychological theorist, originated a hypothesis in the middle of the 20th century that emphasized the importance of the first relationships babies have, namely, those with their caregivers, as the basis for future psychological functioning. These ties usually begin in the earliest months of life and develop through repeated interactions between the

23

infant and her caregiver. Attachment relationships lead us to feel pleasure when our attachment figures are nearby, and they help us feel comforted by the presence of attachment figures when we're distressed. Some types of developmental delays tend to be associated with differences in the attachment relationship, whereas others do not. For example, research has shown that most children with autism or any of the disorders related to autism, as well as children with other developmental disorders, develop strong ties to their caregivers just as typically developing children do, although they may show this attachment in atypical ways, such as seeking out parents but avoiding eye contact with them. This can also be the case for children with sensory, self-regulation, or attention problems. In some cases these signs of attachment, such as seeking to be near parents and caregivers, may also develop slightly later than in typical children. **But without a doubt, most children with ASD and other delays have very special relationships with their parents and other caregivers; they make efforts to be near their caregivers, and they actively seek them when they are distressed.** In fact, the strength of these bonds often means that parents can be their child's most powerful teachers. Like other young children, most toddlers at risk for ASD, attention-deficit/hyperactivity disorder (ADHD), and cognitive delay use their attachment figures, such as parents, as a place of safety and familiarity from which they can venture out and explore their world. They also use their attachment relationship as a place to which they can return for comfort when they are hurt or scared.

From age 6 to 12 months, typically developing children usually use these attachment relationships to develop the ability to engage in back-and-forth social interaction. For children who have been adopted after the age of 6 months, the attachment bond may take a bit longer to form, and spending lots of time together in face-to-face interactions, stimulating and sharing positive affect, should be helpful to this process. Infants and caregivers engage in frequent episodes of face-to-face interaction, many of which happen during the kinds of highly familiar daily routines we talk about in Parts II and III. For example, a 7- to 9-month-old infant sitting in a high chair at mealtime will often watch his caregiver's face, may imitate facial expressions he sees, and will begin to understand his parent's facial expressions. Equally important, the infant will begin to understand that his experience of the world may be different from his parents' experience. Caregivers attempt to teach this to young children by pointing out things that the child may not be noticing. The mother who points to a bird outside the window and, with an excited voice, encourages the child to follow her pointing finger to find the bird is teaching the child that she sees something interesting that the child may not have seen and that the experience can be shared. You can imagine how important this sharing of attention, or "joint attention," might be in learning other things, such as language. When the mom points to a bird and says "Look! A bird!", if the child can see what his mother is pointing to, he can start to learn what a "bird" is and, perhaps even more important, he can start to see his mother as someone more knowledgeable from whom he can learn many things.

Over time the child will begin to make efforts not only to see what the parent is looking at, but also to share her experience with the parent, as she begins to recognize that the adult partner may not be attending to the same things she is noticing. At first infants do this by shifting their gaze between the person they're interacting with and the object of interest. But quickly children learn that pointing is a much more effective way to direct adult attention to an object of interest. Typically developing children usually begin to point between 9 and 12 months, although it can sometimes appear as late as 15 months. Children's use of pointing or eye gaze, and eventually language, to direct another person's attention to an object of interest is another form of joint attention. It is an important achievement in the development of reciprocal social interaction, and it is usually evident by age 1. Joint attention can be initiated by the child by holding something up, by pointing to it, or by looking back and forth from the object to the adult; or the child can respond to the adult's initiating joint attention by following the adult's gaze or point. Both forms of joint attention should be developing by age 1, and both are extremely important.

Children also use their attachment relationships to regulate negative emotions, such as fear, pain, or distress. We talked about this earlier when we discussed children's efforts to find their caregivers when they are hurt or frightened. As they grow older, toddlers use attachment relationships to control their feelings in more subtle ways. Toddlers often look at their caregivers in uncertain situations (for example, when a stranger approaches or they hear an unfamiliar sound), and they use their caregiver's facial expressions to assess the safety of a new situation. When distressed, toddlers find comfort in images or objects associated with their caregivers. A toddler who carries a picture of his mother at daycare or clings to her keys, is trying to use his recollection of his mother to manage feelings of sadness or worry.

We now understand that children at risk for ASD seem to use eye contact less than other infants and toddlers, starting in the first year of life, and, in turn, we understand that not making much eye contact during infancy appears to be a risk factor for an infant's ability to meet social and emotional milestones. That means that children who will later be diagnosed with an autism-related disorder may be less likely to engage in the kind of interactive exchanges we just described. They may be less likely to pay attention to a parent's facial expressions, to imitate these expressions, and to learn to understand them, as well as to imitate simple behaviors (like clapping or blowing raspberries). They are likely to pay less heed to parents' efforts to call something to their attention, and they are much less likely to try to call their parents' attention to something using pointing or gaze shifting (looking back and forth between the object and the parent). Some children at risk for ASD seem to struggle to use images or reminders of caregivers to comfort them when caregivers are not present. Despite having a clear attachment to their parents, children at risk for ASD are less able to use their attachment relationships to develop social interaction skills and other thinking and language skills and to manage their own feelings of distress as they grow older. This can also be true of children with other developmental disorders, such as those adopted from orphanages with poor and inconsistent caregiving.

We can attempt to address some of these difficulties by using interactive exchanges early in development to draw young children's attention to adults' facial expressions, to stimulate the child to feel positive emotion while interacting with parents, to share positive emotion with parents by being happy together, and to begin to understand and initiate joint attention (following the adult's gaze or point and initiating gaze shifting and pointing themselves). Those interactive exchanges, which we describe in more detail in Parts II and III of this book, are designed to help young children begin to use their attachment relationships in a more typical fashion that allows for the breadth of emotional learning that comes from these relationships, despite their neurologically based difficulties with eye contact and emotion sharing. Children with ASD may not seek or use these crucial experiences on their own, as typically developing children do; instead, they require that we direct their attention to these types of activities and actively tempt them to engage with us.

Behavioral strategies rely on the underlying relationship between caregiver and child to teach toddlers patterns of reciprocal exchange. The stronger the connection between a teacher and child, the more likely the child will be to pay attention to that teacher and the more important that teacher's praise and demonstrations of affection and pleasure will be to the child. For these reasons, parents are truly a child's most important teachers. Behavioral strategies also use the child's preferences to guide the selection of rewarding activities used to teach behaviors that are crucial for forming and strengthening attachments, such as eye contact and pointing for joint attention. Using behavioral teaching methods, parents can systematically teach these important behaviors or strengthen them when they are weak. Eye contact and the sharing of experiences using joint attention, can, in turn, strengthen attachment whether attachment emerged naturally in the first year or was explicitly taught and practiced.

BEHAVIORAL TEACHING

Now let's turn to the basic ideas behind behavioral teaching. If you want to learn more about it, look at the Resources section at the end of this book for some excellent books and websites where you can learn more.

Behavioral teaching is based on the science of how children learn. The basic principles apply to adults as well, and also to other animals, but we're going to focus our examples on the things that you might want your young child to learn.

The most fundamental idea is that teachers (including parents) must reward behavior that they want to teach or that they want a child to do more often. Most of the other teaching methods that we will explain depend on this basic idea: Reward the behavior that you want to teach.

Let's say we're trying to teach a child to wave good-bye when another person waves good-bye to her. She knows how to wave but doesn't do it very often or when her mom wants her to. (Later we'll talk about what to do if the child doesn't yet know how to wave.) So her mom decides to work on teaching the child to wave good-bye more often. She begins by making sure that whenever the child waves good-bye to anyone, the other person responds with enthusiasm, giving the child a lot of attention, praise, and maybe even turning his own wave into a tickle by reaching toward the child and giving a little tickle or gentle poke (only if the child likes that, of course). If Mom is holding the child when she waves back, Mom can also give her a little squeeze or tickle, along with praise. For example, Mother might say something like "Yay! You waved bye-bye," or "What a nice girl waving bye-bye," and quickly give the child a little tickle or maybe even a small piece of a favorite treat. The point here is that whenever someone waves good-bye to the child, and she waves back, the result is a lot of fun for her. The reward also gives an extra signal for a child who has difficulty learning or paying attention to emotional signals that that behavior is one she should repeat. Over time, when somebody waves bye-bye to her, she will be more and more likely to wave back.

Most parents reward their children's new behaviors naturally, with a smile, increased eye contact, or a comment, because they are excited to see their child learn new skills. But some children with ASD may not find those things rewarding—or not rewarding enough to establish new behaviors or strengthen existing ones. We will talk later about how to make praise and social interaction more rewarding for children with ASD.

Why We Should Reward Children for Doing What We Want Them to Do

Some people feel a little uncomfortable, especially at first, rewarding their children for doing what they've been asked to do. They may feel that children should simply learn to do what their parents tell them to do and that a reward is not necessary. It would be nice if young children did what we told them to all the time just because it was right, but they often don't! Many, many studies have shown that using small rewards to increase a behavior we want to see from our children (or ourselves) is the most effective way to teach, so why deny yourself, or your child, this route to success?

The idea that learning depends on rewards doesn't apply just to children. It applies to all of us, even though we may not be aware of it. We all learn in this way. If a teacher gives a lesson and her students look interested and pay attention, their response is a reward that encourages her to keep teaching in the same way. If you prepare a meal for your family that they all really enjoy, you are much more likely to make the same meal again because their showing how much they liked it was a reward to you. The approval of people we care about is a powerful reward. Even just the satisfaction you get from knowing you did something difficult is a reward you give yourself. And of course getting paid for a job is a powerful reward.

The point we're making is that all adults and children continue to do the things for which they tend to get rewarded; sometimes the reward is money, sometimes it's approval from others, sometimes it's getting a treat from your mom, and sometimes it's just feeling satisfaction because you did the right thing. Doing things for rewards is just the way our brains are built. And for young children, especially those who don't yet understand a lot of language or pay a lot of attention to adults' approval, something that feels good or tastes good, like a tickle or a treat, may be the reward that works best.

Rewards Given Immediately after a Behavior Can Reinforce It

Anything that a child likes can serve as a reward, but it's important to know that rewards reinforce the behavior that came *just before them*. When a reward is given *immediately* after a child does a certain behavior, and the result is that the child does that behavior more often, we call that reward a "reinforcer" because it has reinforced or strengthened the behavior it followed. When we reinforce a behavior, that behavior is more likely to happen again in the future. In this book we will sometimes use the word "reinforcer" to mean a reward that you give the child right after he does something that you want him to do more often. We can't emphasize enough how important timing is: For a reward to work as a reinforcer it really has to be given *immediately* after the behavior you are trying to reinforce. For example, let's say that your child gives you a bite of her cookie. You are just about to say "Thank you! What nice sharing!" but before you can say that, she throws the rest of her cookie on the floor. If you go ahead and give her the praise, you will risk reinforcing what came just before, namely, her throwing her cookie on the floor!

For some children, praise, approval, or enthusiasm from parents is not an effective reward to start with, because the child doesn't seem to care very much about it. But if we give some small treats that they like *while* we praise them, *or just after* we praise them, then over time the praise can become a good reward by itself, and then we can use it to increase desirable behavior and teach new skills.

So, to go back to our example of getting the child to wave bye-bye more consistently, whenever the child waves back to someone, the adult caring for her will enthusiastically praise her ("Great waving!" or "Yay! You waved bye-bye to Daddy!") and then immediately give her a little tickle (if she likes it) or a small treat, like a small piece of a cookie. In this case, the cookie or the tickle is the effective reinforcer, but after a while, as the child learns to enjoy the praise more and more, the praise alone will serve as the reinforcer.

Take Advantage of Natural Reinforcers

Some reinforcers occur naturally. *Natural reinforcers* are those that happen as a direct result of the behavior. For example, if your child requests something by speaking, pointing, or looking at it, your giving it to her is a natural reinforcer. Or if you offer your child a spoonful of something to eat and she says "no," by speaking, using a gesture, or turning her head away, your withdrawing the spoon is a natural reinforcer too, because you have *taken away* something she *doesn't* want. The next time she is offered something she doesn't want, she will be even more likely to use this type of communication to say no. And if your child has difficulty opening something, like a juice box, and asks for your help using a word or a sign or by handing it back to you with an expectant look, your opening it for her is a naturally occurring reinforcer for her having asked for your help. These reinforcers are very desirable because many people in the child's environment are likely to provide them without really thinking about it, and they are easy to sustain. So when a natural reinforcer "works" for the child (that is, it is rewarding enough to increase the desired behavior), you should use it.

Some toys have built-in reinforcers that teach children to use them correctly. For example, say a child is playing with an animal puzzle and each time she places a piece correctly, the puzzle emits the sound of the animal shown on the piece she has just placed. If she likes that, wants to hear the sound again, and as a result, learns to do the puzzle, the animal sound could be considered a naturally occurring reinforcer of sorts, because it happened automatically as a result of placing the piece correctly.

Other types of reinforcers are not natural consequences of the desired behavior but often occur quite naturally. For example, if your child helps you pick up a toy to put it away, and you praise him enthusiastically and show happy emotion, that might increase the likelihood that your child will help you pick up more toys. If so, that's great, because, again, many people in the child's environment are likely to provide this kind of reinforcement without really thinking about it, so it's easy to sustain. However, many young children, especially those at risk for ASD, need additional reinforcement to get their behavior and skills moving in the right direction. For some children, a big smile, paired with a small edible treat, a tickle with a feather, or blowing some bubbles, immediately after the enthusiastic praise is given, may work better. If you see that your child learns better with the judicious use of reinforcers that are not natural consequences of the behavior, or that do not occur quite as naturally, such as an edible treat, or access to a favorite toy or activity, then by all means use them. Not only will these reinforcers increase desired behaviors, but, over time, as they are paired with social praise and happy facial expressions, they will teach the child who is not instinctively attuned to smiles and praise to attend to and enjoy naturally occurring social rewards.

Phase Out Rewards as the Behavior Increases

Sometimes parents have another objection to the idea of rewarding good behavior; they think the child will come to expect rewards and will never do anything without them. The solution to that concern is to gradually use fewer and fewer rewards as your child learns a new skill and finds it easier and easier. Eventually your child won't need a specific reward each time. Often, using the skill either results in a reward that occurs naturally or becomes part of a chain of behaviors that leads to a naturally occurring reward, or the behavior has become automatic or easy and requires little effort. This happens very often in typical development as well. In toilet training, for example, many parents of typical children provide lots of reinforcement—praise, telling Grandma, going for a treat—for using the toilet successfully. After a while, however, these reinforcers can be phased out, and the successful toileting will become a habit. We generally do this with toilet training because we understand it to be a fairly difficult process that the child may or may not be tremendously motivated to learn. For a child with delays in communication and social skills, things that may come more naturally to other children, such as waving good-bye, may also fall into the same category.

Most of the time you won't need to continue giving rewards when your child practices a skill you have taught her, but even if you do, the child will eventually need only small, occasional rewards. When you are teaching a new skill, or are starting to work on getting your child to do something more often, start with giving her a highly preferred reward every time she does it. The reward can be anything that she really loves, such as a small piece of a favorite cookie or candy, or a spin around in your arms. After she is doing the new skill more easily and more often, try praising her enthusiastically each time, but give her a smaller reward like a little tickle, or use the same reward but less frequently, such as every two or three times. If that goes all right, try cutting back even more, but *be careful to phase out your rewards very gradually.*

Pick Rewards Your Child Really Likes

What rewards should you use with your young child? You should start with things you know he likes, so it's important to think about your child as an individual. What do you know your child likes? Think about that for a minute. It can be a toy or an object he likes to play with. It can be an activity like going on a swing or playing on the playground equipment, playing at a sand table or in the sandbox, or watching bubbles that you blow for him. Some children like rather intense stimulation, or that's what it takes to get their attention, like being lifted high up in the air, bounced fast on someone's knee, a rather enthusiastic cheer or loud music with a fast beat, while others find this kind of stimulation scary and prefer gentle voices, gentle touch, and soothing music. And of course many children like one or the other at different times. Be as sensitive as you can to what your child prefers when he's excited, sleepy, calm, or even bored, so you can use a reward that he really likes and that will work as a reinforcer. Watch carefully to see which toys and activities he gravitates to when free to do as he pleases.

Sometimes the most powerful reinforcer for a young child is a food treat, so think about what your child's favorite foods are, especially if she has foods that she thinks of as special treats. Most children have things they strongly like to eat or drink, so identifying at least a couple of food rewards is a good idea, especially in the beginning. For many children, a sip of juice or another favorite drink works well as a reward. There are a few important points to remember about using food or drink as rewards:

- You should never hold back the basic nutrition your child needs. Always make sure that she gets her basic foods, as well as you can. But if there's a special treat that your child likes a lot but doesn't need to get her nutrition, like a cookie, piece of candy, or potato chip, you can save that treat to use as a reward.

- If you save that treat to use only as a reinforcer, and don't make it freely available at other times, it will work better as a reinforcer.

- You don't have to use large amounts of whatever rewards you offer. In fact, if you use the rewards in very small amounts, your child will probably stay interested in those rewards longer. Remember, we often get tired of the things we get easily or in large amounts. So don't give her a whole cookie as a reinforcer; give her a small piece.

- Be aware that she will probably get bored with a reinforcer if you use it too often. If you see her losing interest, switch to another reinforcer. For example, you might start an activity using small pieces of potato chip for a reinforcer, then switch to small sips of juice, then switch to blowing bubbles or a pinwheel for her. Remember—you have to figure out what reinforcers will work for your child, and you have to notice when they stop working and it's time to try something different.

Use the chart on page 32 to make some notes about reinforcers that might work well for your child, or copy the form or download and print it from *www.guilford.com/ fein-forms*. Next to each potential reinforcer, note if there's a time when it seems to work best. For example, food treats may work best an hour or more after a meal, when your child might be getting a little hungry. Favorite songs might work best when she's getting tired. Being swung might work best when she's awake and alert; swinging her when she's tired might just make her fussy. Notice what your child likes and when and use this information to make your reinforcers as powerful as possible.

One more note about picking reinforcers: Try not to use things your child likes but that will be disruptive or annoying to adults or other children, like turning light switches on and off. Also, try not to use activities or toys that will isolate the child because they are solitary activities that your child tends to do repetitively, like lining up small toys or watching the wheels of a toy car spin. We will talk more later about these kinds of self-absorbing activities, why they are not desirable, and how to encourage more interactive activities to replace these behaviors.

TEACHING A NEW SKILL

Now let's talk about what to do when you want to teach your child a new skill, something he doesn't already know how to do. For example, let's say you want to teach him to imitate you doing a simple action such as raising your arms in the air. You want to give the child a chance to do it so that you can reward him immediately after he does it. But what if the child doesn't know how to do it? Let's say the child doesn't know how to imitate, so you can't just show him what you want—you will have to help him do the action you want him to do. This help or guidance is called a "prompt." The most help would be if you actually physically helped the child do what you are asking him to do. For example, if you say, "Do this," and raise your arms, you might need to show the child how to do it by taking his hands in yours and gently raising his arms. Always be sure to do this gently; you don't want your child to feel uncomfortable while you are prompting him.

If you see that he starts to do what you've asked, then back off and give less help. For example, if you say, "Do this," and raise your arms, and then just touch him on the wrist or under the elbows and give a little push upward and he raises his arms,

REINFORCERS FOR MY CHILD

Food treats	Drink treats	Activities (going on swings, going in the car, bubbles, favorite songs or music)	Toys and books	Sensory or movement (being swung, bounced, tickled)

that's great! He needed less of a prompt. Maybe after a few more tries, just reaching out your arms toward his will be enough of a prompt for the child to imitate you. Always give the least help that the child needs; otherwise he might come to depend on you to prompt him every time. This idea of giving less and less help is called "fading your prompt," or just "prompt fading." Often, children will need many repetitions of the same prompt before being ready to fade to a lesser prompt, so do not expect to fade your prompts *too* quickly, and always give the child enough help for him to be completely successful. As soon as the child does what he is asked, praise him enthusiastically and pair that with another reinforcer as well (or just praise him if he has come to like that). It doesn't matter how much help he needed—you should always reinforce him for doing what you asked, even if he needed a full physical prompt, because behavior that is immediately followed by a reinforcer will be more likely to occur in the future, so you want the behaviors you are trying to teach to be associated with reinforcement. The best kind of teaching gives the child lots of chances for success, even if he needs the prompts to be successful for a while. It's better to show him the right way to do something and then gradually fade out the help. That works much better than letting him do it the wrong way and then trying to correct the mistakes.

Teaching an Action That Has Several Parts

Now here's the last important point about behavioral teaching that we're going to cover here: What if what you want to teach is not something simple, like raising arms, but something a bit more complicated? You might think waving bye-bye in response to another person's wave is simple, but it actually has several parts to it— and you have to figure out what the different parts or steps are. You can do this by doing it yourself, very slowly, and paying attention to all the steps you have to do. Here's an example using the behavior of waving bye-bye:

1. Look at the person waving to you.
2. Raise arm.
3. Wave (wiggle fingers or move hand from side-to-side).
4. Put hand down.

Although there are actually four steps; look, raise arm, wave hand, put arm down, two of those steps, raising the arm and moving the hand from side-to-side, can easily be taught as one step. And in all likelihood, the child will naturally put his arm down after he waves. So, in this case, you really only need to teach the child two steps; "Look" and "Wave."

1. First, we want the child to look toward the adult who is saying good-bye and waving. We'll ask that adult to say good-bye with enthusiasm from pretty close by and loud enough to be sure the child can hear him so that he is likely to get the child's attention. Then we try to catch the child looking at the adult, and once she does that, the adult should praise her immediately and give her a small reward like a tickle with a feather or maybe by turning the wave into a tickle. For children who

tend not to look directly into other people's eyes, the adult may want to wave his hand close to his own eyes at first as this can work as a prompt to help the child look at the adult's eyes. We call this making eye contact, and we'll talk a lot more about this throughout the book. Because this adult is the only person who can really tell if the child is making eye contact, he should be the one to praise and reward the child. It may take several sets of practice trials for the child to learn the step of looking at the person who is waving to him, and that's okay.

2. Once she is doing that with good consistency (meaning not all the time, but most of the time), we add the next step: the wave. This time, as the child looks at the person who is waving to her and saying bye-bye, we will prompt her to raise her arm and move her hand, followed immediately by praise and/or a reward. You will probably not have to teach her to lower her arm, as she will probably do this naturally.

Remember, at each step, use the smallest prompt you can. It's easy for children to come to depend on our prompts and not to learn to do the skill by themselves, so our job is to reward the child for more and more independence in doing the skill. But we do it slowly, gradually reducing the amount of help we give. This can require a lot of patience on your part!

PUTTING IT TOGETHER

Behavioral strategies rely to some extent on an underlying relationship between caregiver and child or between teacher/therapist and student. If the child is attached to the caregiver and relies on him or her for comfort, fun, safety, and having needs met, reinforcers given by that person may be more effective. (In fact, many parents may be able to teach their own children using social reinforcers like smiling, laughter, hugs, or praise, before the child's therapists are able to because of this powerful relationship.) Good behavioral teaching uses the child's preferences to guide the selection of reinforcing activities and things (like toys or treats), tuning in to the child's feelings, and ensuring that they enjoy the experiences you are providing. In addition, a good behavioral teacher is joyful! The best teachers are overflowing with fun, enjoyment, and obvious affection for the children they teach, and they communicate these feelings with warmth and humor. This is a very powerful way to stimulate feelings of attachment.

On the other side of the coin, social interaction can usefully incorporate and be strengthened via behavioral methods by directly reinforcing behaviors, such as eye contact, which support social interaction. Much of what a good behaviorist is trying to reinforce and build is exactly what attachment theory tells us are foundational skills for optimal social development: eye contact, nonverbal communication through facial expression, shared enjoyment, joint attention through gaze and pointing, and attention to the caregiver's language. In this book, behavioral teaching and stimulating feelings of attachment are both front and center.

CHAPTER 3

12 Rules to Play By

Now that we have explained two of the most important general approaches to teaching toddlers at risk—fostering attachment and using behavioral principles—we're going to move on to some very important, more specific points to keep in mind when teaching and playing with your toddler. In Chapter 4, we describe the things you want your toddler to learn. With those pieces in place, you'll have the full foundation for using daily routines to stimulate development in your child through play and be ready for Parts II and III, where games and activities designed to teach these things are described.

1. START EARLY

In Chapter 2, we talked a lot about why it's so important to teach your child to be more tuned in to adults and about some general ways to do that. This focus on increasing social interactions (and eye contact in particular) and helping the child learn to enjoy adult company and find it fun is important throughout childhood, but it's *especially* important when your child is very young and is just setting off on her developmental pathway.

Think of it this way: You're the captain of a ship leaving New York for Europe, and you're heading in a slightly wrong direction. If you wait until you're close to the shores of Europe and make a slight change in the angle of your direction, you will make only a slight adjustment in where you arrive. But if you change course near the beginning of your trip, you'll make a big difference in where you wind up.

Children respond to the activities we describe in this book in different ways. Some of their reaction depends on the biology of their brains. In other words, some

35

children begin life with greater neurological deficits than others, and the magnitude of these biological deficits affects how responsive the child will be to teaching. Even though some children are more capable of learning quickly or making bigger changes than others, whatever changes they can make are more likely to be brought about by intervention very early in life. So it's a good investment to put in the time and energy as soon as possible. Don't let professionals or other parents tell you to wait and see what happens with your child's development. If you're concerned about your child's development, and especially about the way she relates to adults, you should start doing the types of activities we describe in this book as early as you can. Even if your child's development turns out to be completely typical, these activities will be fun and educational.

2. USE FUN ACTIVITIES TO DISTRACT A CHILD WHO IS TOO SELF-ABSORBED

We don't want any child to be wrapped up in his own little world, thinking his own thoughts; engaging in repetitive, stereotypic movements or play; talking to himself by repeating scripts from TV shows, songs, and books; or looking at inanimate objects for extended periods of time and ignoring other people, which is what we often see in toddlers who are at risk for ASD. When a child tends to remain engaged in self-absorbed activity, and often seems far away from the adults taking care of him, it can be tempting to let him just do that for several reasons: it allows the adults to get their own chores done, the child is not demanding attention, or the adult may have seen the child become upset when these activities are interrupted and might think the child somehow *needs* to do what he is doing. This is a mistake. The more you allow the child to stay wrapped up in his self-absorbed activities, the more he will stay involved with them.

What you want to do is to take every opportunity to get the child's attention, make yourself a source of fun, and make interacting with you so enjoyable that you'll be able to compete with the interest he finds in those solitary activities. We understand that you will have things to do around the house, or work you have to get done, but it's really important to spend as much time as you possibly can, or have other warm and responsive adults spend as much time as they can, getting the child to interact with others in a pleasurable way. Some children are easier to distract from these self-absorbed activities than others. For a child who is very hard to distract, you may not always succeed, but even if your successes are limited, every minute that he is engaged with you is an opportunity to learn skills and increase attachment.

We'll show you some ways to distract the child from his own self-absorption. Many therapists call this self-absorbed activity "stereotypic behavior." It includes things like

- staring at lights, shadows, or water;
- twiddling fingers near the eyes;

- flapping arms and hands (especially when the child is not particularly excited);
- rocking, pacing, or running back and forth;
- doing things over and over (like throwing small objects behind furniture, turning lights on and off, opening and closing doors or drawers);
- lining up toys or objects and getting down to look at them at eye level;
- tensing of limbs and facial grimacing; and
- flipping or twirling small objects and watching them fall to the ground.

Some of these behaviors can be hard to distinguish from normal toddler repetitive behavior. Toddlers often like to do the same thing over and over or be read the same book over and over in the same way. They may flap their arms when excited. However, if your instinct tells you that your child is doing these things in an unusual way, or if he does these things in a solitary way that does not encourage you to join him, you may want to interrupt these activities. You never want to scold your child or punish him for this self-absorbed behavior; you want to distract him and engage him in something that is more fun. For example, we recently watched a talented therapist with a 2-year-old who was holding a transparent scarf up to the light and staring at it in that self-absorbed way; the therapist took the other end of the scarf and began a game of peekaboo with the scarf, drawing the child's attention to the game and to herself, and soon had the child enjoying a social interaction.

Sometimes imitating what the child is doing will get his attention, and this is a good thing to try when your child is playing with toys or singing a song he likes or is engaged in pretty much any behavior that you could do together. Just make sure the child is interested in your imitating him. If he's ignoring you, imitating him will be pointless. However, it's best *not* to imitate these self-absorbed, stereotypic activities. Examples of these kinds of self-absorbed activities would be lying on the floor and watching the wheels of a toy car go back and forth repetitively or flapping a piece of paper in front of the eyes over and over again.

Using the same toy or material, like the car or the piece of paper, to create a fun experience that you and the child can share together can be a good way to encourage a child to interact with others rather than remain self-absorbed. In the case of a child watching the car wheels, a good idea would be to interrupt and redirect that behavior by pretending to make the car race with another car or speed down a surface that is set on an incline. In much the same way, if the child is flapping a piece of paper in front of his face, you could use it to play peekaboo; or you could make a paper airplane with it and have fun with your child making it fly it through the air and chasing after it. If your child is flapping something soft and wiggly, you could tickle him with it or put it on your head in a funny way.

- *If your child is pushing buttons on an electronic toy or a sound book, try making a funny action for each different button.* For example, when he presses one button, you might dance; when he presses another, you might tickle him; when he presses another, you might pretend to fall down. Hopefully he will begin to press the buttons and look at you expectantly, preparing to laugh at your antics! If the game catches on, you might be able to turn the tables and press the buttons to have him do the funny actions.

- *If your child loves to open and close cabinets, you might try turning his game into a treasure hunt by hiding a special item in one* ("Is the teddy in here? No. Is the teddy in here? Yes!").

- *If your child enjoys throwing toys over his baby gate, you might sit on the other side and try to catch them with a basket,* cheering loudly when you catch one ("He shoots, he scores!") and hamming up your disappointment when you (purposely) miss ("Oops!"). Hopefully your child will begin to enjoy this game and you will stop needing to try to "catch" the objects and instead will be able to put down the basket and join him, turning it into a target game. You could begin to place baskets farther away and take turns throwing toys toward them.

You can use a general rule of trying to get your child's attention at least once every 20 seconds while you're playing with him; unless you have to be busy else-where, don't let him go more than 20 seconds without having some kind of social interaction, even if it's very brief.

Some children at risk for ASD also seem to enjoy lining things up, like little toy animals or cars. If this is the case with your child, try to do other things with the same toys. For example, put on some music and pretend the animals are danc-ing together or set up a small track for the cars or the animals and pretend they're racing. One very creative mother used her child's obsession with lining up empty soda bottles to create a bowling game, where they lined up the bottles together and took turns rolling a beach ball to knock them over. She used lots of praise for taking turns with the ball, or knocking down lots of bottles, and made it extra fun by increasing the suspense ("Here it goes . . . here it goes . . . CRASH!! Okay, my turn!"). The interactive game was then more fun than the self-absorbed activity. If you find there is no way to turn a repetitive behavior into a social game, you might simply want to limit access to it, for example, by placing tape over the light switches that he can reach and likes to flick on and off or by putting certain toys away for a while, such as cars with wheels that a child tends to spin repeatedly. The important thing is to interrupt and redirect this kind of self-absorbed behavior whenever you see it, especially if it is very repetitive. The goal in all of these examples is to distract your child from the repetitive, solitary activities and increase your child's engage-ment with other people, especially YOU!

3. USE NATURALLY OCCURRING INTERACTIONS AND ROUTINES

The use of naturally occurring routines to teach many of these skills is important for several reasons. First, it allows us to begin with a routine, which the toddler already knows and finds comfortable and familiar. We can enter that activity without disrupting it and then *shape* the routine to incorporate new skills and behaviors. This can be a routine involving mealtime, bathtime, bedtime, or any regular activity. Second, the toddler can learn new skills in many situations throughout the course of her day, and learning new skills in varied, real-life situations helps to promote what we call "generalization." When skills are generalized, children tend to use them more and are better able to use them in new situations and with different people; there is less danger that a child will use her new skills only in interaction with a specific partner or only in a specific context or location.

The use of natural routines also allows us to provide many opportunities to practice new skills. In addition to the few hours of focused instruction, which might be provided by a therapist, parents can teach, demonstrate, and support the development of new skills as part of their natural interaction with their child throughout her day. If your child is getting a few hours of focused instruction from a therapist, you can greatly expand her learning opportunities by using these activities throughout the day. **Definitely consult with your child's therapist, if she has one, to see which skills are being targeted and get advice about which areas of learning might be most helpful to focus on.** In learning social skills, like language, imitation, and nonverbal communication, as in learning many other tasks, frequent practice helps children learn skills more quickly.

Last, but certainly not least, parents often report that incorporating interactive routines into their daily caregiving activities helps create the frequent positive interactions that they so desire with their young children and that are so important for the child to experience. Over time, these interactions may provide the child with more opportunities to laugh and smile with her caregivers in shared enjoyment, which will reduce any stress she is experiencing, increase her emotional expression, and most important, support the strengthening of her attachments to others, which may in turn help the development of more complex interactions and social skills.

If your child has a professional interventionist who is conducting more intensive teaching sessions, you should still take advantage of the naturally occurring learning opportunities that you can provide throughout the day and evening in the context of everyday routines; they will greatly enrich what you can teach your child and how often she gets to practice her skills and learn to expand the types of joyful interactions she can share with you.

4. CHANGE ROUTINES IN A FUNNY WAY

Once a child has learned a routine, mix it up by doing something different and unexpected. He'll probably find that surprising and funny, and therefore it will get his attention. For example, you could try putting only one inch of water in the bathtub, or use a slotted spoon to feed soup, and when you get his attention, make a fuss about it: "Oh, Mommy is so silly! She forgot all the water!" or "Mommy is so silly. That spoon won't work." This not only will help direct the child's attention to what you're doing but may also help to develop his sense of humor.

5. LEAVE OFF ENDINGS

One technique is to leave off words at the end or in the middle of something and let the child fill it in. For example, during dressing, you could say, "Sock is on. Sock is off!" (as you quickly sweep it off), using a rising intonation and drawing out the word "is" to get your child's attention and eye contact, and create suspenseful anticipation. Then, "Hat is on. Hat is . . . off!", while you're putting the hat on and taking it off. Then you could say, "Shoe is on," while you put it on, then, "Shoe is _____," with a questioning tone of voice as you take it off. If the child attempts to say "off," give enthusiastic praise and repeat a few more times with other pieces of clothing, each time rewarding any attempt to say "off" with praise and maybe a tickle if your child likes it. Of course, the tickle is just an example. Use whatever reinforcers (rewards) your child likes.

You can do this technique with many simple concepts, like "in" and "out" (e.g., using a scarf in a paper towel tube), "open" and "shut" (e.g., using an umbrella) going "up" and "down" (e.g., building up blocks and knocking them down). See the list of words in Chapter 17 for additional words and concepts.

Songs also work very well with this procedure. If there's a song your child likes and has heard many times, you can leave off the final word, or a familiar word in the middle, and reward her for filling it in. If the child doesn't fill it in, wait 3 or 4 seconds to make sure she's not going to fill it in and then fill it in yourself. Some children have very good memories and are great at this even if they are not sure what the word they are saying means, so if you can tie the word the child is filling in to something in the environment, all the better—for example, "Five little monkeys [then both of you jump as he says 'jumping'] on the _____ [and you can point to the bed as he says 'bed']. One fell off and bumped his _____ [touch your head or his as he says the word 'head']."

6. HELP THE CHILD INCLUDE OTHERS IN PLAY

When playing with your young child, you want him to include you in some way, even if it's just by looking at you. If your child already knows how to imitate, you may find that he'll imitate you if you play right next to him with the same materials. Sometimes just playing with the same toy next to your child, switching back and forth between imitating his play and demonstrating new ways to play that he may not have thought of, is enough to get him to switch his attention between his play and you.

Sometimes we think we're playing well with children if we sit next to them and narrate their actions—for example, "Now you're spinning the wheels. Now you're making the car go." But this does not encourage back-and-forth interaction. **When playing with your child, try thinking, "Could he be doing the same thing if I were in another room?" If the answer is "Yes," you may have to work a little harder to make sure he's checking in with you and paying attention to your facial expressions and actions.** For example, if your child is playing with a toy, and he goes more than a minute or so without checking back with you, you could say, "My turn," and gently take away his toy and put it on your head with a big smile or do something else with it that's fun or silly. When he looks at you, give it back to him and say, "Your turn." Or you might try being the "keeper" of the toys. For example, when using Play-Doh or doing a puzzle, you may have to keep all the cookie cutters or puzzle pieces behind you or in your lap so that he has to look at you or point whenever he wants one.

7. GET YOUR CHILD'S ATTENTION BY USING WHAT SHE LIKES

You can begin by noticing the situations in which your child pays the best attention to you. Is it when you remove distractions and engage with her in a quiet space? Is it during games that involve a lot of movement or sensory stimulation, such as when you're swinging her, bouncing her up and down, rolling her up in blankets, or playing with her in the water? Is it when you engage with her in new activities, or is it more with familiar activities?

Some children want to be social but find it overstimulating and uncomfortably exciting, so it helps them if you create an environment without a lot of distractions or make your interactions more predictable. For example, some children like to be hugged, kissed, and picked up only when they have a little bit of warning that they are about to be touched (for example, "I'm going to pick you up on the count of three. One, two, three!"). Other children may need a lot of excitement to pull them away from their own interests and tempt them into social interaction. To make yourself interesting to the child, and to make sure you have her attention, you may have to exaggerate—use big gestures, exaggerated facial expressions, and vary the pitch and volume of your voice. This will get the child's attention and also help her understand what you're trying to communicate. The brains of infants and toddlers are developing at a remarkable rate. Your child is learning every hour that she is awake. **Your goal is to have her learn about social interactions for as much of that time as possible. That means setting up situations in which she attends to you best, as often as possible throughout her day.**

Watch your child as you move through the day with her.

- Is there a particular toy she likes?
- Does she like taking a bath with or without bubbles?
- Does she light up when she sees the family dog?
- Are there particular foods she likes?
- Does she like loud music, or does it make her fearful or uncomfortable?
- Does she like lotion on her arms and legs, or does she try to pull away?
- Do new things help her pay more attention, or do they overwhelm her?
- Does she like dark or cozy spaces like forts or tents?

- Are there certain kinds of touch she loves or dislikes?
- Does she like being lifted up high or bounced on your lap, or does that make her uncomfortable or scared?

Using activities, foods, and objects that your child likes is very important in helping you get her attention. Using these objects and activities will provide lots of opportunities to help her feel more attached to you, to learn skills, and to spend less time in self-absorbed thoughts and activities. For example, if your child likes lotion, you can use it to teach body parts by labeling body parts as you put lotion on. If she likes a tickle better than the lotion, you can use a feather or soft brush, like a make-up brush, to tickle her and label the body parts as you do so. Remember, however, that using what the child is interested in doesn't mean letting her remain engaged in self-absorbed activities; it means tempting her out of these activities by getting her attention with objects and activities you know she likes or is interested in.

If your child doesn't seem interested in a toy or activity, don't give up immediately—sometimes a couple of repetitions of the invitation to play, in an animated way, may be all you need to get her attention. But if she is really not interested, move on to another activity.

8. HAVE THEME DAYS

Another good way to teach a concept is to have a theme for the day.

- *Any color can be a theme.* For example, have "red day" where you both dress all in red, eat lots of red foods, point out all the red things at the grocery store, play with lots of red toys, make an art project at the dinner table with just red paint or red crayons or red Play-Doh.

- *Or any animal can be a theme.* You could have your "word of the day" be "fish," where you go to an aquarium or pet store to look at fish, cut out aluminum foil fish for the bath, eat goldfish crackers for snack, and go to the library and read books about fish. If your word of the day is "caterpillar," read *The Very Hungry Caterpillar,* make a caterpillar out of an empty egg carton, catch a caterpillar outside and place it in a jar with dirt and leaves to observe for a while, wrap yourselves up in blanket "cocoons" and pretend to emerge and flap your wings flying around like butterflies, and sing "The Fuzzy Caterpillar" to the tune of "The Itsy Bitsy Spider." ("The fuzzy caterpillar curled up on a leaf, spun her little chrysalis, then she fell asleep. While she was sleeping she dreamed that she could fly, and later when she woke up, she was a butterfly.") If your word of the day is "dog," visit a dog, make a "doghouse" for a stuffed dog out of a cardboard box and decorate it with dog stickers, read *Doggies* by Sandra Boynton, sing "How Much Is That Doggie in the Window?", and play "Doggie Doggie, Where's Your Bone?" (You need at least two people in addition to the child for this game. The child hides her eyes, one adult hides a toy behind his back, and everyone chants "Doggie Doggie, where's your bone? Somebody took it from your home. Upstairs downstairs from the telephone. Wake up doggie and find your bone." [If your child's attention span is very short, just use the first line.] The child then uncovers her eyes and guesses who has the toy behind his or her back.)

- *A favorite food can be a theme.* For example, if your child likes eggs, you can cook and eat them in various ways, color them, hide plastic eggs for your child to find and collect in a basket and put little treats, pictures or notes in some of the eggs, read and act out "Humpty Dumpty," hatch "grow eggs," visit a chicken coop, or find a bird's nest or a picture of one and point out the eggs to your child.

- *You can create seasonal themes* by having a flower day in the spring, leaf and pumpkin days in the fall, and a snow day in the winter. In the spring you can find and pick flowers, make cut-out flowers, or read books about flowers. In the fall, you can take a trip to a pumpkin patch, sing "Five Little Pumpkins Sitting on a Vine," cook pumpkin seeds or pumpkin pie for a snack, play "hide the pumpkin" or "pass the pumpkin" (pass it back and forth as quickly as possible until music stops), and make pumpkins by coloring paper plates orange. In the winter you can play in the snow, catch snowflakes, make snow angels, bring snow inside and melt it, and read *A Snowy Day.*

- *You can also just do what you normally do, but change things up a tiny bit to match your theme day.* For example, if your word of the day is "dog" read some picture books about dogs. If you normally hide something in a sandbox, you might hide dog bones or little dog figures in the sandbox that day. You might change up the words to the song you normally sing (e.g., sing "The Dog Went over the Mountain," instead of "The Bear Went over the Mountain"), pretend to be a mother dog and her puppy when you snuggle, and when you read bedtime books, make sure to draw special attention to any dogs you see. Repeating the same concept over and over again in a very short period often helps a child understand the concept more quickly.

9. TEACH SKILLS AT OR JUST ABOVE YOUR CHILD'S CURRENT LEVEL

Figure out what your child knows or knows how to do and focus on teaching skills that are just above her current level, but not too far above. For example, if your child has no words or gestures, you will want to teach simple signs (like "help" and "all done"; see Chapter 17) or simple words or word approximations (like "baba" to request or label her bottle) as the next step. If she has simple signs and gestures and some sounds but no real words, you can focus on teaching her to understand and say just a few words, like "eat" and "juice" and "mama." And if she has many words but no word combinations, you can focus on teaching some simple word combinations, like "want Cheerios," "want juice," or "all done eating." When you are teaching children to say words, it is a good idea to begin with the words for things your child likes a lot so that she can ask for them. That is because asking for things she likes a lot will be especially motivating for her, so she may try very hard to say those kinds of words.

It's best to spend some time working on skills that are about on your child's level (like teaching additional single words if she already has some words) and some skills that are just above her level, but don't frustrate her and yourself by trying to teach things that are months or years ahead of where she currently is.

The same principle could apply to the words you use to speak to your child. If she says "juice," you could say "more juice" or "yummy juice" or "red juice." If she says "more juice," you could say, "You want more juice. Here you go." You are using language that is just a little more advanced than what your child is saying.

10. DO NOT ENCOURAGE INDEPENDENCE TOO SOON

It may seem a bit strange to actually encourage your child to be dependent on you, but when children are slow to learn about social interactions we want to give them as much practice as possible. It can make day-to-day life easier when we have a child who is very independent at an early age—a child who may like to play by himself, who does not keep asking for things, and does not demand a lot of attention—but this is not necessarily a good thing. To help the child increase his enjoyment of adults, and attention to adults, it helps if the child *needs* adults, not only for basic things like food and clothing but also for entertainment. So when possible, use toys that require an adult's help, like balloons and bubbles, or blocks for stacking and knocking down. Think about removing toys that encourage the child to play by himself, like toys that he can easily make spin or light up. And you can encourage the child to ask for help, in whatever way he can, by putting toys and snacks in clear containers that he cannot open or in places that he can see but not reach. If he says any words, you can prompt him to ask for help by modeling the language for him ("need help?"), or gently helping him point to what he wants while you put yourself where he can easily see you and make eye contact, and then immediately help him get the thing he wants.

Many electronic devices fall into the category of toys that can be socially isolating. Children can learn many things from iPads and similar devices, and of course, sometimes, you absolutely have to get that dinner cooked; but that being said, when the child is on the iPad, he is not learning to engage with other people, which is priority number one.

11. INVOLVE OTHER FAMILY MEMBERS

It will benefit your child if there are other adults or an older sibling who can do some of these activities with her, such as a second parent, another relative, a babysitter, or close friends. This will help the child establish other close relationships and learn to carry over the feelings and skills you are encouraging. Playing games and doing routines with more than one person should help to promote generalization of the skills your child is learning; practicing skills with different adults will help her to be more flexible with those skills and to use them more often and in different kinds of situations. Other adults or older siblings can also do some of the fun activities and keep the child socially engaged when you are not available.

If there is a sibling or other close family member around the same age as your child, or within a couple of years of your child's age, it's helpful to involve the other child in the play at the same time. The benefit of giving the two children the same thing to play with at the same time is that, if your child can imitate others, she will have a nice model for age-appropriate play. If she does not yet imitate others, you could prompt her to do some of the same things with the toy that the other child does and then praise her for doing that. Ideally, she will discover that she enjoys these new ways of playing with her toys. Sometimes even children who are not especially interested in paying attention to adults will be interested in paying attention to other children.

12. DON'T FORGET THE BEHAVIORAL PRINCIPLES YOU JUST LEARNED

While teaching your child and getting him interested in interacting with you, don't forget to use the behavioral principles we discussed in Chapter 2. When he doesn't participate in games with you, or imitate you, or watch what you're doing, prompt him to do these things—not necessarily all the time, but most of the time. For example, if you're playing a game or singing a song where you're both supposed to clap, you can gently take your child's hands and help him clap. If he is not looking at you or making eye contact with you, you can prompt attention and eye contact by putting yourself right in front of him or holding up a favorite treat near your face. And then, when he does what you want, whether he needed prompting or not, be sure to give him enthusiastic praise and whatever else he likes, such as a tickle or a bounce on your lap, or maybe even a small piece of a favorite treat. Prompting and immediately rewarding the desired behavior will make it more likely that the behavior will occur next time.

CHAPTER 4

Language, Eye Contact, and Imagination

IMPORTANT TARGETS OF LEARNING

In the last two chapters we talked about general strategies for teaching your child new skills. Now we're going to discuss the most important things you want your child to learn at this early age. We describe six important targets of learning in this chapter. In Part II, where we describe teaching games that you can use for toddlers during specific daily routines, we tell you which learning targets each one is designed to address.

ADULTS ARE FUN, REWARDING, AND COMFORTING: SOCIAL ENGAGEMENT

As we said earlier, the single most important thing you want your toddler to learn is that adults are important, rewarding, and fun to interact with. You can tell when a child feels connected to adults because he will seek them out, smile when he sees them, reach for them or go to them when he is happy. Also, when the child is frightened, sad, hungry, or hurting, he knows that the important adults in his life can make him feel better, so he finds them comforting as well as fun and wants to be with them when he is unhappy. When children feel connected to and interested in adults, they want the adults who are special to them to pay attention to what they're doing. And children enjoy showing things to adults and look forward to the adults' reaction. When an adult and child look at each other, we say they're making eye contact. Eye contact is such an important part of social engagement that we've made it a separate teaching target and will discuss it more in a minute.

One way to think about what young children are learning is to divide it into two sets:

1. *They're learning how things work.* The child has to learn that, when he holds something and lets go of it, it falls. If it's made of glass, it breaks; if it's made of cloth, it doesn't. If you hide something under a blanket and then take the blanket away, the thing is still there. Most children pay attention to objects and how they work and do not have special trouble with this kind of learning, although some children learn more slowly than others.

2. *They're learning how* people *work.* This second set of things is just as important. Children have to learn that other people are just like them—they have feelings, they think and remember, they do things based on how they feel and what they want. A child must learn to understand and use language by listening to other people. He also needs to learn how to look at things from another person's point of view. For example, if he knows that his little sister is hungry, and Mommy puts a cookie on the table, he should be able to predict that his sister is likely to take the cookie and eat it.

If a child is very interested in objects, but not in people, he may not learn this second set of things at all or will learn them very slowly and not very well. So the most important thing for the child under 3 years old, and for older children who don't have these skills, is to pay good attention to you and other people, so he can learn how people work and enjoy being with people. Therefore, you should concentrate on getting your child to enjoy being with you, to pay attention to you, and to listen to your voice, even if he doesn't understand very much of what you're saying. You do this by making yourself the source of fun and comfort, by reinforcing (rewarding) your child for paying attention to you and communicating with you, and by adjusting your language and nonverbal communication so he's likely to understand what you're trying to communicate to him. If your child is often very absorbed in his own thoughts and activities, maybe in doing unusual little things over and over, and doesn't pay a lot of attention to other people, try to get his attention gently whenever you can. Put yourself where he will see you, do fun things to him and with him, to get his attention in a way that will be pleasant for him. This will reinforce him for paying attention to you, for doing what you ask, and for initiating communication with you.

The more he pays attention to you, the better. But this is very important: Don't try to get his attention by yelling at him or doing something he won't like, because you want him to learn that adults are pleasant to be around. You don't want him to pay attention because he's afraid of adults. At the same time, you can also teach some skills, but do it without a lot of pressure, in a gentle, gradual way and while you're doing the natural everyday activities like dressing, feeding, bathing, and playing. **The most important skills that a child of this age learns are connecting and communicating, which, for a young child, means paying attention to what you're saying and how you're feeling and trying to let you know how he feels and what he wants.**

While most of the ideas and suggestions in this book are designed to teach the child a variety of skills in the context of everyday activities, an even more important aspect of this kind of teaching is simply that it increases the amount of time the child spends actively engaged with others. For this reason, teaching the child to pay attention to the important adults in his life is a good place to start.

A closely related thing to work on is to **stimulate happy feelings** in the child. Many toddlers at risk for ASD and other developmental disorders don't show a lot of happy feelings on their face, especially when they are interacting with others; they don't often seem happy and bubbly, and sometimes their emotion seems flat, although this is not always the case. For a child who doesn't show a lot of positive emotion, it's important to stimulate a variety of positive emotions whenever possible, by doing things that make him smile or laugh. You also want him to connect these happy feelings with the important people in his life. Furthermore, children at risk for ASD, even older children, sometimes have an especially difficult time understanding the language of emotions or labeling what they are feeling, so another thing to work on is to help them know what they're feeling. One way to get started with this is to imitate a child's facial expressions and label the emotion for him.

EYE CONTACT

Eye contact is a particularly important part of social interaction. One way we'll show you to get more eye contact is to use eye contact as the on/off switch for having fun. For example, say you're standing in front of your child on a swing, which she likes. You catch hold of the swing and push it the way she likes it, a few times. When your child is not looking at you, catch hold of the swing and hold it still, waiting for eye contact. As soon as your child looks at you, immediately give her another push just the way she likes it. Do this repeatedly, so that whenever she looks away, you stop the swing and then resume pushing her the instant she reestablishes eye contact. You can do the same thing with many other toys, especially toys that your child cannot play with easily all by herself. Bubbles, tops, and pinwheels are especially good for this kind of play, and music works well too. You can play music electronically or sing to your child; if your child is enjoying the music and looking at you, keep the music or singing going. When she looks away from you, pause the activity until she looks into your eyes. As soon as you have eye contact, begin again immediately. You can add a word or two if you like as well, and by keeping your language simple and using only key words, like "Blow" or "Sing" or "Ready, set, go!" you may be able to teach some language at the same time, or at least introduce your child to some new words.

You can also make it easier for your child to make eye contact with you by kneeling in front of her so that you appear closer to her height (see the drawing at the top of page 49). You don't have to be exactly eye-to-eye, but if you're close enough and just in front of her she will see you right away when she looks up, yet you won't be so close that it's unpleasant for her.

Another teaching technique you can use for a child who really avoids looking you in the eye, which we mentioned in Chapter 3, is to hold a favorite treat just in front of your nose, as shown in the drawing at the bottom of page 49. When the

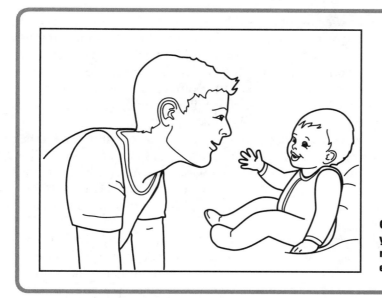

Getting down to your baby's level makes eye contact easier.

child looks up at it, her gaze will likely take in your eyes as well. As soon as she establishes eye contact with you, praise her for nice looking and give her the treat. If she doesn't make eye contact, you can slowly move the treat closer to your eyes until it's just in front of your eyes. Either way, remember that holding the treat so close to your eyes is a prompt and, ultimately, you want your child to make eye contact with you naturally, without a prompt. So, over time, as her spontaneous eye contact increases, try holding the treat farther and farther away from your eyes, and then try calling her name without using the treat to prompt eye contact. Just hold it in

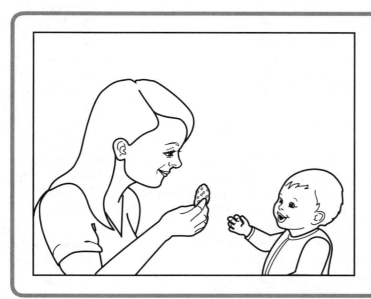

Encourage eye contact by holding a favored treat in front of your nose.

your hand with your hand closed around it so that it's out of sight, wait for her eye contact, and then produce it with a flourish while saying, "I have something for you!" Also, you certainly don't need to give your child a treat or even praise her every time she makes eye contact with you. In fact, once she begins to respond to you with eye contact, and to initiate eye contact more often on her own, it's better to reinforce eye contact more naturally—for example, telling your child she has beautiful eyes, winking at her, or just giving her a big smile.

BUT—here's an important thing to keep in mind. We don't want to imply that your child should be looking at you all the time. That would be unnatural. To get a sense of this, observe other babies and toddlers with their parents and see how often they look at each other, especially how often babies and toddlers look at their caregivers while they're playing with them or engaged in another activity such as mealtime or diaper changing.

Of particular importance is the toddler's sharing of experiences with her caregiver by alternating eye gaze between a parent and the object(s) of her interest. This is sometimes referred to as joint attention or shared attention. When a baby or toddler is reading a story with a caregiver, for example, you should see her shift her gaze between the pictures in the book and the caregiver's face. When you see a toddler in the market or shopping mall with a parent, or at a place that's novel or interesting for the child, like the park, the beach, or the zoo, you should see this sharing of attention very often.

If you have a baby or toddler who is not making good eye contact, use the activities in this book to increase eye contact by using it as the on switch for fun. (In Part II, we identify activities that are especially good for working on this.) When you get eye contact, and then the child looks away, let the fun activity continue for a short time without requiring your child to look back at you. If your child has not returned her gaze to you by the time you feel it would be natural for her to do so in the context of this activity, stop the activity and put yourself in front of the child, requiring eye contact to start again.

It's hard to specify exactly how many seconds the eye contact should last or how long to go without it before prompting it again, because this will vary from activity to activity and will also depend on how many other points of interest there are in the environment at the time. For example, if you're sitting face-to-face with your child, feeding her, and talking to her, and there are minimal distractions in the room competing for your child's attention, you should expect her to look at you for periods of about 3 to 8 seconds while she is chewing and swallowing, after which she'll probably glance at the bowl of food and watch the progress of the spoon for a few seconds before establishing eye contact with you again. On the other hand, once your child's hunger is satisfied, especially if there is another person, or perhaps a pet dog or cat in the room, your child may naturally begin to divide her attention between you and the other objects of interest, giving you a bit less eye contact than when you were first feeding her and that's fine.

If you're someplace new, or particularly exciting—for example, the zoo or a toy store—and the child is very interested in what she's seeing, you should expect her to check in with you frequently, making brief periods of eye contact and sharing a smile with you or perhaps checking to see where you're looking, but there will likely be much longer periods during which she's attending to the new things in her environment and not engaging in extended periods of eye contact with you.

Still, we can't emphasize enough the importance of eye contact in the social development of infants and toddlers. So while we don't want you to force your child to make constant eye contact with you, we do want you to encourage frequent, prolonged periods of eye contact that assure you of her engagement with you and feel natural in the context of the activities you're doing together.

NONVERBAL COMMUNICATION

We're also going to use daily activities to help the child develop simple communication skills, like requesting to be all done with an activity, requesting to continue an activity, requesting a toy or snack, and choosing between two things. When children don't have simple words or gestures to request these things, they tend to just whine or cry. It's very important for them to learn that there are simple and effective ways for them to communicate with the adults taking care of them. This is especially important for children who don't yet have language or those who struggle a great deal to learn language. Sometimes people get the idea of communication confused with the idea of language. This is because most people do use language to communicate. However, children who don't yet understand words, as well as those who can't yet speak words, can still learn to communicate very simple messages using only eye contact and gestures such as pointing, shaking the head to communicate no, nodding to communicate yes, smiling to show pleasure, frowning to show they don't like something, or using a sign like holding the arms up, palms facing in, and then turning the hands at the wrist so that the palms are facing out to communicate "all done" (shown below).

Communication of messages using only eye contact, facial expression, and gesture is often referred to as "nonverbal communication" because, although words are helpful, they are not necessary for this kind of communication.

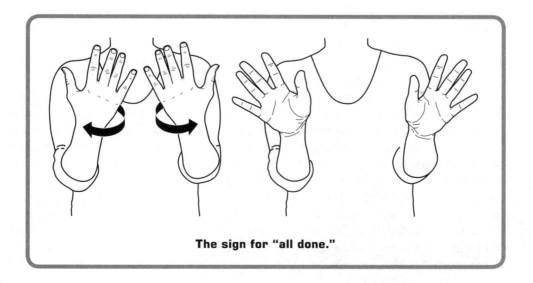

The sign for "all done."

LANGUAGE

In addition to teaching basic nonverbal communication, as you move through your day with your child, there will be many opportunities to teach language in a fun way. When we talk about teaching language, we're referring to both speaking and understanding language. This means we'll be giving you lots of ideas for how to teach your child to understand words when he hears them spoken by others as well as to begin to say words himself.

Very young children like, and learn better with, repetition, so you might want to make a list of simple words to start with (not too many—maybe start with just five to 10 words) and find chances throughout the day to use them. You can look at the list of words and phrases in Chapter 17 to get some ideas. This doesn't mean that you won't work on many, many more words throughout the day; however, we're suggesting that you choose five to 10 words that you'll focus on and keep in mind throughout the day so you can look for opportunities to use them in ways that will help your child learn them. We'll show you lots of examples of this all throughout Part II of this book. Saying what the child is doing can be very helpful in teaching language; for example, you might say, "We're eating! Yum! Eating Cheerios." But, just like imitating what the child is doing, he must be paying attention to you for this to be effective. If you're just commenting on what he's doing, and he's not paying attention, he won't learn any language, and he might actually learn to tune you out. **So make sure you have his attention, put yourself close to him to make it easier for him to pay attention, and don't talk too much!** If you repeat yourself frequently, it will become easier for your child to tune you out. Instead, try to *say things only once* and make sure you have your child's attention *before* you speak to him. The best way to gauge this is to determine whether he is looking at you and, if not, to make sure you have his eye contact before you begin to speak. And if you ask him to do something, like, "Come here," say it only once. If he doesn't respond within 3 to 5 seconds, prompt him to do as you've asked and praise him for doing it, even if you had to help him.

When adults talk to very young children, they often use exaggerated up-and-down speech (you can practice while you say "Up, up, up! Down, down, down"). This exaggerated tone is good at getting babies' and toddlers' attention, so don't hesitate to use it, even if you feel a bit silly at first. If your child is a bit older, but not yet talking very much, this exaggerated tone will still help him learn language. Very young children also like simple melodies, and like to hear them repeated, so don't be shy about singing silly songs or saying nursery rhymes to your child. You can even make them up if you're so inclined. This is a great way to introduce your child to simple language.

Remember how we said you could use eye contact as the on/off switch for a fun activity? You can do this using language and gestures too. If you think your child is ready to learn to say some simple words, you can teach him to say words using this idea of reinforcing the words he says by immediately doing what he has asked of you. This should really show him how powerful his words are! For example, if your child likes to be tickled, you can teach him a little routine by saying "I'm going to give you a tickle, tickle, TICKLE!" Each time you say the word "tickle," move your fingers in a tickle motion. Move your hands a little closer to him each time you say the word "tickle" and also say the word a little louder each time, drawing out the suspense. The third time you say the word "tickle" is when you actually tickle him. Make it as fun and suspenseful as you can! Once your child becomes familiar with this routine, you'll probably see that he's paying special attention to you just before the third time you say the word "tickle." When you see him doing this, try to pause and look at him expectantly. See if he fills in the blank and says the word himself. If he does, or even tries, give him the best tickle ever! If not, you can try to prompt him by asking him to "Say 'tickle'" or by giving him the first sound: "t." Because speech is difficult to prompt, if he doesn't follow your prompt, just pause for a moment and then start over, continuing as you were doing it before, where you are the one saying "tickle" all three times and then tickling him. Keep doing this fun routine, and try to check now and then to see if he will fill in the blank, by pausing before you say the word "tickle" on the third try. If he isn't quite ready to begin saying words, be sure to reinforce any nonverbal attempt he makes to communicate with you. For example, he may lean toward you or reach his hands out toward you after the second time you say the word "tickle," and this will show you that he is engaged and excited about what's coming next. **Either way, you're still teaching him that interacting with you is a lot of fun, and this is the most important lesson of all.**

IMITATION

Imitation is a wonderful foundation skill. If a child can imitate your actions, it will be easier for her to learn to pretend, to learn words, and to learn skills such as waving, feeding herself, dressing herself, making a puzzle, or throwing a ball. Throughout the day, you can demonstrate very simple actions such as raising your arms to show the child what to do while you're dressing her (see the drawings below). When

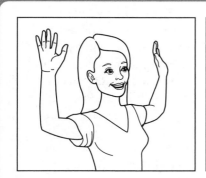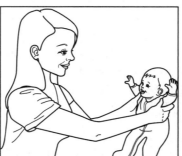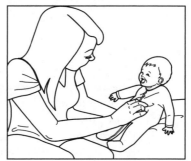

Help your child learn simple actions like raising her arms through imitation.

you have her shirt ready to put on, raise both of your arms in the air and say, "Arms up," in a happy tone of voice. If she imitates you, give her enthusiastic praise and blow a raspberry on her belly or do something else she likes before putting on her shirt. If she does not try to imitate you, help her by gently taking her hands and raising them upward. Then praise her just as if she did it all by herself. Try again a few times before putting on her shirt. If you do this every time you get your child dressed and undressed, it probably won't be long before she begins to imitate you when you put your arms up.

PRETEND PLAY

Another important thing to work on is helping your child start to understand and enjoy pretend play. You can do this by demonstrating very simple pretend, like pretending to drink from a cup the child can see is empty, or pretending to feed a baby doll or a stuffed animal during meal or snack times. Or, just before bedtime, you can help your child put one of his dolls or stuffed animals to bed and give it a kiss good night! When you do these things, be sure to show your child that pretend play is fun and that you're enjoying pretending things with him.

Here's another way to introduce the idea of pretending to your child: If something provokes a strong emotional reaction in your child, either positive or negative, do an "instant replay" with a doll to help the child understand what happened and help him understand the idea of pretend. For example, if he fell and bumped his knee and cried, after he feels better, you could act that out with a doll, having the doll fall and cry, then kissing the doll's boo-boo and helping the child kiss the doll's boo-boo, applying a Band-Aid, and saying, "Now he feels all better." If Mommy's glasses fell off when she sneezed and you both laughed, try replaying this with stuffed animals or dolls. Capitalizing on the child's strong emotional reactions will help him learn the idea of play pretend more quickly.

As we go through the daily routine activities and games in Part II we'll label each one with the target(s) of learning that it helps teach. These will include the targets we described in this chapter—social engagement, eye contact, nonverbal communication, language, imitation, and pretend play—and some activities will also target general "thinking" skills, like understanding that similar things can go together or that when something disappears from sight it still exists. In a few places, we will also list "behavior," which refers to getting the child to cooperate in situations like cleaning up or staying with you in the supermarket. For Part III, in the chapters on babies in the first year of life, the targets of learning are described in the beginning of each chapter; for example, for the first 3 months of life, you want the baby to learn that he is safe, that he is loved, and that people are important to pay attention to.

As you read about activities you can weave into parts of your day, remember these are just suggestions. Try adapting them for other parts of the day and don't hesitate to make up your own games and activities. You're the best person to figure out what your child is ready to learn and what kinds of activities your child likes.

PART II

GAMES AND ACTIVITIES FOR TODDLERS AT RISK

CHAPTER 5

Waking Up
and Going to Sleep

Waking up and going to sleep happens every day, and for most toddlers, at least twice a day, giving you lots of opportunities to do some of these activities. It can also be a very cuddly time, both when they are waking up and as they are winding down and preparing for a nap or bedtime. **But**—children can also be quite cranky during these times, so be sure to tailor the stimulation you provide and the behavior you're trying to elicit to the child's mood. Keep the stimulation quiet and soothing and keep your demands very simple.

 ## 1. GOOD MORNING, ELMO! LANGUAGE

Morning or nap wake-up time can be a great time to get in lots of repetitive language practice. When you lift your child out of his crib or bed, carry him around the room, stopping to greet some of his favorite stuffed animals, dolls, action figures, or pictures of family members and say good morning to each of them. For example, you could say, "Good morning, Elmo, good morning, Teddy, good morning, Doggie, good morning, Grandma [if you have a picture of her], good morning, Grandpa," and so on. If you do this every morning or nap wake-up time, and your child becomes familiar with this routine, you can try to use the filling-in procedure (see Chapter 3) to see if you can get your child to begin trying to say the names himself. For example, walk up to the picture of Grandma and say, "Good morning, _____," and then pause and look at him with an expectant look and see if he says "Grandma" or even makes the "g" sound. If he does, cheer for him and give him a big squeeze or whatever demonstration of affection he likes best. If he doesn't fill in the word, you can try prompting by saying, "Good morning [pause for

57

a second or two], Gra . . . ," and see if he completes the word. If he does, give him enthusiastic praise, a squeeze or tickle, or whatever you think he might like. If you think "Granny" or "Grandma" is too hard, think up another word for Grandma using sounds you know he can make, like "Gaga" or "Buhbuh" or "Ganny." If you think there's another word he might be ready to say, like "doggy" or "teddy," try that one instead. If he is not ready to fill in with words or sounds, that's okay. It's important just to keep letting him hear these words, so continue doing the greeting routine and exposing him to this language.

One Note about Waking Up

Some children are very groggy and sleepy for a few minutes after waking up, and it takes them a little while to be really awake. If your child is hungry, give him some milk or juice from his bottle or cup so he will not be too uncomfortable to pay attention. If he's cranky, try to soothe him and let him settle down. You can carry him around the room and do your greeting routine, but don't expect him to try to talk until he is really awake. The exact routine will depend on your child's habits, but you might try something like this: lift him out of the crib, sit with him on your lap for a couple of minutes while he's waking up, give him a small bottle or cup of milk if he's hungry, *then* walk around and do the greeting routines; once with *you* doing all the talking, and then a second time when he's more awake, leaving off names for *him* to fill in.

 ## 2. NIGHT-NIGHT, DADDY!   LANGUAGE/SOCIAL ENGAGEMENT

Nighttime (or going down for a nap) is also a great time to get in more repetitive language practice and to become more aware of each important person in the house. The goal is to have your child give good night kisses or hugs to any of her family members and favorite dolls or stuffed animals and to practice hearing, and maybe saying, their names, before she goes to bed. Make up a routine for saying good night at bedtime similar to the one you use for morning greetings. For example, you could carry her around to each family member, saying, "Kiss Daddy. Night-night, Daddy. Kiss brother. Night-night, brother." (Of course, in this case, you would use the brother's name.) If you think your child is ready, try using the filling-in procedure to see if she will fill in with a name.

When you say, "Kiss Daddy," you can lean her in so that she's close enough to give Daddy a kiss, and Daddy should give her a comfortable hug and kiss. Prompting a kiss can be difficult, but Daddy's kiss will serve as a model, and you can gently prompt her to give Daddy a hug by raising her arms and putting them around him. When you carry her to her bed for bedtime or nap, continue the routine by carrying her around her bedroom and saying good night (or "night-night") to dolls, stuffed animals, or pictures. Walk around the room and stop in front of your child's favorite stuffed animals to give *them* good night kisses and hugs and say, "Night-night, teddy bear." And she can collect a few stuffed animals along the way to take with her into the bed. If your child is cranky or fussy because she's very tired, keep the routine short and try to soothe her with whatever works for her—singing a favorite song, nursery rhymes, cuddling, reading a favorite book, lying in bed with her favorite stuffed animal while you read or sing to her.

3. UP, UP, AND AWAY!

LANGUAGE/NONVERBAL COMMUNICATION/ SOCIAL ENGAGEMENT/EYE CONTACT

Waking in the morning or after a nap is also a great time to get in some practice with the word "up." When you walk in and see your child standing in his crib, give him a warm, delighted smile to show him how happy you are to see him. Then reach out your arms and say, "Up?!" in a happy, *questioning* or rising tone of voice. If he doesn't raise his arms, then use a gentle physical prompt to raise his arms in a gesture that means "Pick me up" or "I want up." Then immediately pick him up and give him a warm hug and a nice cuddle. Picking him up is a natural reinforcer because you are providing just what he is asking for. Make sure you have his eye contact just before you lift him out of the crib, even if it's very brief. To get eye contact, put yourself right in front of him where it's easy for him to look at you. If he doesn't look at you, put yourself right where he's looking, just before you pick him up. Do this often when he wakes in the morning as well as when he wakes from his nap. Before long, he should be raising his arms on his own and looking right at you when he wants to get out of his crib.

You can also use this idea during any part of the day when you have a spare minute. Suppose your child *loves* when you pick him up and swing him around. To teach him to understand the word "up" you can say, "Up?!" in a happy, questioning tone of voice and then immediately use a physical prompt to raise his arms in a gesture that means "Pick me up" or "I want up." Then immediately pick him up and swing him around, reinforcing his request to be picked up (even if he needed a prompt to do it). Repeat this several times in a row. Then on the third or fourth try, say, "Up?!" just as you did before. But this time, don't use a physical prompt to raise his arms. Instead, just wait for a moment and look expectantly at your child. If he raises his arms at all, even only slightly, pick him right up and swing him around again, saying something like, "Up, up, and AWAY!!!" In this way his "up" gesture becomes the "on switch" for the fun. If he doesn't raise his arms, just prompt him again by gently helping him raise his arms and then continue as before for a few more tries. You can try fading your prompt gradually too. For example, you can try to prompt him by reaching down to him as if you are about to pick him up and seeing if he raises his arms. If he does, great! Pick him up immediately and swing him around if he likes that. If not, go back again to a physical prompt, delaying your prompts from time to time until you see that he is beginning to do it by himself. If you do this every day for even a few days, your child may soon learn to raise his arms when you say, "Up? Want *up*?" Or, "Do you want *up*?"

If he is able to imitate sounds or words, you can also try to work on having him say the word "up" just before you pick him up. Simply reach your arms toward your child as if you are about to pick him up and say, "Say up." When you do this, it will be important to put the emphasis on the word "up" and to deemphasize the word "say." Do this by saying "say" quickly and softly, pausing briefly, and then opening your mouth wide and saying the word "up" more slowly, using a clear, slightly louder tone of voice. Make sure there is a noticeable difference in volume between the very soft "say" and the very clear "up." This should help to increase the likelihood that your child will understand that when you ask him to "say" something, you want him to repeat only the word or words that come *after* the word "say."

4. THE BLANKET GAME   SOCIAL ENGAGEMENT/LANGUAGE

Another activity that many children enjoy a great deal is being taken for a ride on a blanket. You can make a game of it by taking a blanket to your child, having her sit on it on the floor, and pulling the blanket, and her with it, around the room. Do it slowly so she doesn't fall off; speed up a bit if she likes it, but try to go at the speed she likes. Stop periodically and prompt her to say "go." You can do this in several ways—by saying, "Go?" or by prompting her with the initial sound "g" or by saying, "Ready, set, go," before you start pulling, eventually using the filling-in procedure to see if she will fill in the word "go." Once she becomes familiar with the "Ready, set, go" routine, simply prompt by saying, "Ready . . . Set . . . ," then pause and see if she fills in with "Go!" If she doesn't yet say any words, you can prompt her to make a sign for go before pulling her some more. See if your child can imitate you making the sign for "go" shown below—you hold both of your index fingers straight up and then move them downward as if pointing with two hands in the forward direction.

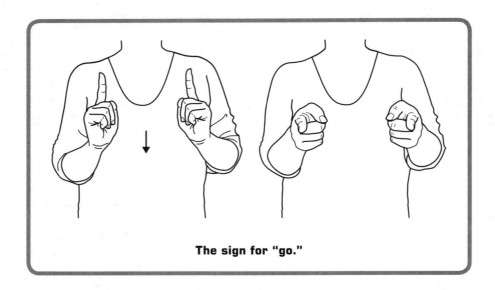

The sign for "go."

If your child has difficulty making this sign, you can make up your own sign for "go," such as a one-handed point or a fist held up over the head. Anything will do! In any case, as soon as your child attempts to communicate the word "go," you should immediately take her on a little ride, then stop again and say, "Ready, set, . . ." or "Ready, set, g . . ." and see if she will make the sign or fill in "go" or "g" another time. If she does, be very excited and say something like, "Go! You said go!" as you pull her. If she doesn't say "Go," just pause for a couple of seconds and fill it in yourself—"Go!"—and then pull her. If you do this at bedtime, you'll want to do a couple of relaxing, calming routines, like reading a book or singing some songs, so that she isn't *too* excited when it's time for her to go to sleep.

5. LET'S GO FAST. LET'S GO SLOW.

LANGUAGE/NONVERBAL COMMUNICATION

Once your child starts saying "g" or "go," you can add the words "fast" and "slow." Pull him around several times very slowly, saying, "Slow . . . slow," and be sure to draw out the word "slooooow," saying it slowly and calmly, then speed up the blanket ride as you say "Now we go FAST!" (only as fast as he enjoys), saying "fast!" quickly in an excited voice. Making your voice sound different when you say the two words heightens the contrast between the two concepts. You can use the filling-in procedure by saying, "Now we go slow," and then speed up and say, "Now we go . . . ," and see if he will attempt to say "fast." You can also ask him to make a choice by saying, "Do you want fast or slow?" If he doesn't yet say words, you can ask, "Do you want fast?" and if he looks at you, or wiggles, or nods, or in some way indicates that that is what he wants, say, "Okay, FAST!" and pull him quickly. Again, going fast is a natural reinforcer because you're providing just what he's asking for. This can be done with other activities as well. For example, when taking a walk, you might hold hands and say "fast" and begin to run fast, and then say "slow" and begin to walk slowly. Or when giving your child a stroller ride or a piggyback ride, you might try the same thing, saying "slow" and walking or pushing slowly and then saying "fast!" and walking or pushing fast.

6. LIGHTS OUT!

LANGUAGE

You can work on the concept of light and dark, as well as the names of different rooms, by walking around the house and turning out the lights in various rooms together just before bedtime. As you enter a room with your child, turn on the light if it's not already on and say, "Now it's light." Then as you leave the room, turn off the light and say, "Now it's dark—good night, kitchen." You can do the same thing in any room. For example, "Now it's dark—good night, bathroom," or "Now it's dark—good night, living room," and so on. And, of course, as your child becomes more and more familiar with this nighttime routine, you can pause at various points and see if she fills in the blanks. If she does, with the correct word or some attempt at the word, be very enthusiastic. You might say, "Kitchen! That's right! It's the kitchen. Good night, kitchen." If you think your child is ready to start saying these words but is not saying them yet, you can prompt her; for example, "Good night, ki . . ." If she doesn't respond correctly, you complete the word for her: "Good night, kitchen." If she does, of course, praise her enthusiastically and give her a little squeeze or a tickle or whatever you think she might enjoy.

7. BEDTIME STORIES

LANGUAGE/SOCIAL ENGAGEMENT

Reading bedtime stories each night is a wonderful routine for any child. Most books work well as naptime stories too. There are so many positive aspects to this routine, but most of all, if the child enjoys this time with you, when you are snuggled up together reading his favorite stories, it will help him look forward to bedtime or naptime, rather than try to delay them. And he will be able to go to sleep feeling calm and safe.

For children who have difficulty learning language, it's a good idea to choose books that use a repetitive language approach to teaching new words. *Brown Bear, Brown Bear* by Bill Martin, Jr., and Eric Carle and *Goodnight Moon* by Margaret Wise Brown are two classic repetitive language books, but there are many others, like counting or alphabet books or books by Sandra Boynton. If you read the same three or four books to your child over and over again, and your child enjoys them, you can try pointing to a picture and pausing before you say the word to see if he'll fill in the blank with the missing word. If you think he might be able to say the word but needs a little help, you can try prompting him with the first sound of the word, like "Good night, mmm . . .'" or "Brown b . . ." Let him see your face while you're making these sounds, too, especially if he can imitate movements.

After you read *Goodnight Moon,* you could keep it going for a minute or two and make it even more fun by holding a flashlight, turning out some of the lights, and shining the flashlight on different parts of the room while saying things like, "Good night, crib; good night, books." Your child may really enjoy being the one to shine the flashlight beam on things he wants to say good night to, or to shine the flashlight on something and have you say good night to the object.

Before you begin reading, try holding up two different books to see if your child will reach for one. Then reinforce by saying, "Oh! You want *Goodnight Moon*! Great!" For the child 9 months and older, you might gently try to shape her fingers into a point as she reaches for her preferred book.

8. HOMEMADE BOOKS

LANGUAGE

If your child likes books, try making your own books, designed especially for her. You can create books to help her learn about herself and her world. There are many, many possibilities. Here are a few examples using the repetitive language approach that we've been talking about.

Names of Foods

If you want to teach your child the names of her favorite foods, you could take pictures of those foods (or download and print images, or even make colored drawings) and make a book called *What Does Baby Eat?* Every other page would be a picture of your child with the words "What does baby eat?" Of course, you would substitute your child's name for the word "baby." Then on the opposite page would be a picture of one of her favorite foods, with the words "Baby eats" and then the word for the food pictured on that page. So, for example, if your child's name is Maggie, the book might read, "What does Maggie eat? Maggie eats bananas." "What does Maggie eat? Maggie eats yogurt." "What does Maggie eat? Maggie eats cereal." "What does Maggie eat? Maggie eats ice cream." "Yum!" All you need to do is take a few 8″ × 11″ sheets of white paper, fold them in half, turn them sideways, and there's your book!

This book would provide a great opportunity to work on the names of foods, as well as the word "eat" and the child's name. Once your child becomes familiar with the book, you could try pausing at various points to see if she fills in the blanks with some of these words. Prompt her with the first sound of the word while you point to the picture; if she doesn't try to say the word, finish it for her. If she does try, be very enthusiastic, even if her try isn't very good. For example, if you say, "What does Maggie eat? Maggie eats . . ." (pause and point to banana) and she says, "ba" or "na," say, "That's right! Maggie eats BANANA!" You are demonstrating the correct way to say the word, but, more important, you are reinforcing with enthusiasm her attempt to say the word.

Names of Clothing

You could also make a book called *What Does Baby Wear?* to help her learn the words for clothing. That book could have pictures of her in her pajamas, swimsuit, coat, and so on, or just pictures of the clothes themselves if that's easier. Read it the same way, pausing occasionally to see if she will attempt to say the word.

Names of Family Members

And you could make a book called *Who Loves Baby?* to help her learn the names of her family members. One page would say "Who loves baby?" and the opposite page would have a picture of Grandma and the words "Grandma loves baby!"

Action Words

If you want to begin teaching your child some action words, you could make a *What Does Baby Do?* book that could have pictures of her eating, drinking, sliding, swinging, sleeping, bathing, reading, and so on.

Information about Your Child

You could even make an *All about Baby* book that could have basic information about your child, like her name, her age, the people in her family, and the things she loves. The possibilities are endless.

If your child does not like books, try first introducing interactive books (you'll probably have to buy these!) that have flaps, pop-ups, or sound buttons. If there are characters she likes or things she is fascinated with, like fish or trains or Elmo, try books about those things. You can buy these or make your own with pictures from magazines or that you download from the Internet.

In any case, keep the bedtime books happy and light. You always want your child to go to sleep thinking happy thoughts!

 ## 9. REMEMBERING THE DAY: HAPPY MEMORIES

LANGUAGE/THINKING

As you sit with your child at bedtime, remind him of the most special parts of his day: "You saw your friend today" or "You went down a big slide today" or "Grandma and Grandpa came to visit you today." If you have a cell phone that takes pictures, and can take a few pictures each day, show them to your child at bedtime to help him remember the happy things about his day. And be sure to remind your child that he felt *happy* to spend time with Grandma and Grandpa and that they were *happy* to spend time with him! If you can get a picture of the child smiling or laughing, or one of the adults or other children smiling or laughing, be sure to show this to your child and say, "Grandma's happy!" Keep it simple—don't remind him of more than about three things. When it's bedtime or even naptime, the morning activity might be only a distant memory to your child!

 ## 10. LULLABY AND GOOD NIGHT

SOCIAL ENGAGEMENT/
NONVERBAL COMMUNICATION

Just before it's finally time for your child to go to sleep, sing her a lullaby. Music is very soothing for bedtime, especially if you sing the same set of songs every night. You might even make three pictures to go with three different lullabies; for example, you could make a star for "Twinkle Twinkle Little Star," a cradle for "Rock-a-Bye

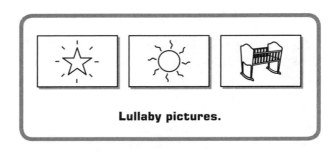

Lullaby pictures.

Baby," and a sun for "You Are My Sunshine." Point to the picture that goes with the song you're about to sing. Then you can ask the child to request a song by putting all three pictures on his crib or bed and help him point to the picture of the song he wants or hand you the picture and then sing the song he requested. If he points to a picture but then doesn't like the song you start, put the picture back on the bed, help him point to a different one, and try singing it. Once he learns which picture stands for which song, always sing the one he requests, even if you're getting very tired of it! The idea is to teach him to request what he wants, and you reward that behavior by giving him what he has requested.

CHAPTER 6

Dressing, Undressing, and Diaper Changing

Dressing, undressing, and diaper changing are routines that also occur multiple times a day and provide lots of great opportunities for teaching and for having fun with games. Since the child is likely to see the same types of clothing each day, they can be very useful for teaching language (like "sock" and "shoe"), concepts (like "hello" and "good-bye"), and object permanence (when Mommy hides behind my shirt, she is still there).

 1. HELLO–GOODBYE **LANGUAGE/PRETEND PLAY/IMITATION**

Diaper changing is a good time to work on some repetitive language routines. You can help the child understand that "hello" signals something or someone new coming into her environment and "good-bye" or "bye" or "bye-bye" (whichever you prefer) signals something or someone leaving.

Saying Hello and Good-Bye to the Child's Clothing

When you take off the wet diaper, say, "Bye-bye, diaper," as you throw it in the trash or diaper pail. When you throw wet pants in the laundry, say, "Bye-bye, wet pants." When you take out dry pants from a drawer, say, "Hello, dry pants." If it's time to change into pajamas, put the clothes you take off into the laundry basket or put them away and say, "Bye-bye, pants; bye-bye, shirt." Make it a fun activity by letting the child throw it into the laundry hamper or by holding it over the hamper, saying, "Bye-bye, shirt," and then "Ready, set," and then pausing before "go" to create suspense about when you're going to let it go. Then say, "Hello, pajamas" as you take them out

66

of the drawer. For an extra dose of silliness, you can say, "Hello, elbow!" as you bend your elbow or he bends his and then, "Bye-bye, elbow" as you straighten your arm or he straightens his. "Hello, knee; bye-bye, knee" often gets just as many giggles.

Saying Hello and Good-Bye Using a Stuffed Animal or Doll

Then you can give a teddy bear or doll a diaper change or a change of clothes using the same words. For example, you could say, "Hello, Teddy! Do you need a diaper change?" and then put a paper towel diaper on Teddy, wet it with a little water, and say, "Teddy needs a new diaper. Bye-bye, wet diaper," while you throw away the "diaper" or have your child throw it in the trash, then put on a dry paper towel "diaper," saying, "Hello, dry diaper." If your child is having fun and you think she might enjoy trying to put a diaper on Teddy by herself, then pour a little water on the new diaper and say something like, "Look! Teddy's wet again!" Then ask your child to change the diaper and throw away the old one, helping her if she needs a little help. Of course, if she doesn't think this activity is fun, move on to something else. If she tries to change Teddy's diaper, give her whatever help she needs and a big reinforcer (praise, tickle, swing, treat) for helping.

Saying Hello and Good-Bye to Objects

You can reinforce this idea with anything you use and then throw away. For example, when taking out a tissue, say, "Hello, tissue" and then say, "Bye-bye, tissue" when you throw it in the trash, or say, "Hello, juice box" when you take it from the refrigerator and then say, "Bye-bye, juice box" when you throw it away. If your child has a pop-up toy or a jack-in-the-box, you can say hello when the characters appear and good-bye when they disappear back into the box or behind a door. When you're cleaning up toys at the end of the day, you can say good-bye to them as you put them away; for example, "Goodbye, block!" each time you drop a block into its box.

Saying Hello and Good-Bye to Other People

Be sure to also reinforce these hello and good-bye concepts with people, so when Daddy or Grandma appears, make a big fuss: "Here's Daddy! Hello, Daddy!" "Here's Grandma! Hello, Grandma!" And when they leave, similarly: "Grandma's going in the car. Bye-bye, Grandma." If you give your child lots of practice at hearing hello and bye-bye, this will make it much easier for her to grasp the idea.

2. THE PEEKABOO GAME   EYE CONTACT/SOCIAL ENGAGEMENT/THINKING

Peekaboo is a great game for working on eye contact and social engagement any time of the day. But if your child is still in diapers, you can use the diaper change as a brief opportunity to play peekaboo. Most children find it fun to see someone pop out from behind something, and you want your child to have lots and lots of experiences with you that are fun. When your child is lying on his back ready to be changed, you can play peekaboo from behind the diaper when you pull it out of the box or the drawer. Hold it up in front of your face (while keeping one hand on your child if he's squirmy) and say in a questioning tone, "Where's Mommy?" Wait just a second, and then pop out from behind the diaper, saying, "Here's Mommy!" or "Here I am!" Try to pop up in front of the child, to make it easier for him to look at your face and your eyes (but not so close that you scare him). You can repeat that a couple of times, especially if the child enjoys it, unless you have a very squirmy child, in which case you should get on with the diaper change! (Or turn the squirming into a game; see Activity 4.) In addition to encouraging eye contact, helping the child enjoy being with you, and perhaps tolerating the diaper change a bit better, peekaboo helps children understand the idea that when something goes away, it doesn't stop existing. This concept is called "object permanence."

 ## 3. STICKY, WET, OPEN, CLOSE   LANGUAGE

Pick a few additional simple words to work on, like "sticky," "wet," "open," or "close." Give your child as many opportunities as you can to hear these selected words in situations that make their meaning clear. For example, let the baby feel the "sticky" tabs on the diaper while you say "sticky" or let her touch a piece of tape while you say "sticky." Let her feel a "wet" wipe from the box while you say "wet" each time you change her diaper. Wash your hands after you change her diaper, and while your hands are still wet, touch her hands and say "wet."

Most children like to throw things in the trash. When the dirty diaper is rolled up and ready to be thrown away, point to the diaper pail or trash bin and say, "Open," and then prompt her to lift the lid of the trash bin or diaper pail by gently putting your hand over hers. Once the lid is open, say, "Bye-bye, diaper," while you prompt her to throw it away by guiding her physically to pick up the wrapped-up diaper and let it go into the trash or diaper pail. Let your child be the one to "open" the trash bin or throw the wet diaper into the trash, telling it "Bye-bye," and later, "Bye-bye, diaper!" or eventually, "Bye-bye, wet diaper!" Be sure to reinforce her attempts to participate in this activity with praise or something else she likes.

Give your child practice with the word "close" by telling her to "close" the trash bin or diaper pail and then prompting her to close the lid if she doesn't do so on her own (reinforcing this even if she needed a prompt with praise or a big "Thank you!"). You can do the same thing after you take clean clothes out of the dresser if you have a dresser drawer that she can reach and that is easy to close (but watch those little hands!).

Your child will pay best attention to you during these times if she can predict and understand what is happening and, ultimately, play a role in the routine. So try repeating these routines and language every time there's a diaper change so that your child gets used to them and begins to understand more and more of the language you're trying to teach her. And remember to praise her and even cheer for her when she does as you've asked.

4. THE DIAPER SONG   LANGUAGE/SOCIAL ENGAGEMENT

Making up silly songs for routines can be a great way to hold your child's attention and increase his enjoyment in being with you. An easy song would be something like this, sung to the tune of "Frère Jacques": "Baby's diaper, baby's diaper, now is dry, now is dry! Now let's take the old one, now let's take the old one, and say bye-bye!" If you let the child throw the old diaper in the trash or diaper pail, this would be a great song to sing just before you hand it to him so that he can toss it in. If you want him to open the trash or diaper pail, ask him to "Open, please," and then be prepared to prompt him to do what you've asked of him and then reinforce him enthusiastically using the word "open" again. You could say something like "Yay! You *opened* it! What a helpful boy!" Some adults feel silly making up and singing songs like that—don't worry about it! Your child won't think it's silly; he'll think it's fun!

For a child who squirms a lot during diaper changes, see if you can turn it into a game. For example, sing "Do the Dipey Dance" or play music for a minute as he squirms and as you do a silly dance yourself and then say, "Now stop!" and stop the music or singing and quickly stop dancing, making yourself "freeze" for a second, and if he stops too, quickly change that diaper. If your child finds this fun, pretty soon that diaper squirming may become a regular 1-minute dance party, with the two of you imitating each other's rhythm and sharing a laugh or smile.

5. RED SHIRT OR BLUE SHIRT?   LANGUAGE/NONVERBAL COMMUNICATION

Letting your child make some choices about what she wears will serve several purposes:

- It might make her more cooperative and easier to dress.
- It will help her learn the names of clothes and colors, as well as other kinds of descriptive language (such as stripes, polka dots, soft, long, short).
- It will help her learn how to communicate what she wants.
- The more choices you give a child, the more she develops a sense of self. (We all define ourselves in part by our choices. "I like to wear purple, I like to swim, I like to listen to country music . . .")

You can put two shirts on her bed or on the floor and say "Do you want to wear the red shirt or the blue shirt? Do you want to wear these pants or these pants?" She can communicate her choice by reaching for the item, by pointing to it, by labeling or describing it ("the red one"), depending on her level of communication skills. If she doesn't make a choice, hold the two shirts very close to her and see which one she reaches for or touches. Regardless of which one she chooses or how she makes the choice, be enthusiastic: "You picked the red one! Okay. We'll put on the red one." Be sure to honor her choices, even if the outfit might not be the one you would have picked!

6. DRESSING MR. TEDDY

PRETEND/IMITATION

Dressing a Doll after Waking Up

When your child wakes up in the morning or from a nap and you're getting him dressed, let him do the same thing with a doll or a stuffed animal. Many such items can be quite difficult to put on; try to use doll clothing that's easy to put on. For example, you could use a teddy bear shirt that slips on the arms and opens in the back. Old baby clothes sometimes work well as doll clothing because they are often sized a little larger than doll clothing and tend to be soft and easy to manipulate. After you put on the child's shirt, you can say, "Now let's dress Mr. Teddy." Hand him the shirt and help him put it on and then have Mr. Teddy thank him enthusiastically.

Putting Teddy to Bed

You can do the same with going to bed. Before you put the child in his bed or crib, say, "Time for nap. Let's put Mr. Teddy down for his nap. Look how sleepy he is. [Pretend to yawn for Teddy.] Let's cover him with his blankie and sing him a song." Help your child do the simpler actions, like covering Teddy with a blanket, and praise him: "What a good mommy/daddy you are. You put Teddy to sleep."

Teaching Imitation with Teddy

You can also practice imitation. Using two dolls or stuffed animals, you can demonstrate putting on or taking off a shirt or pajamas, putting the animal to bed, covering it with a blanket, and as you're doing this, help your child imitate one or more of these actions with *his* doll or stuffed animal. Again, praise him for taking good care of Teddy or doll.

7. SOCK ON, SOCK OFF!

SOCIAL ENGAGEMENT/LANGUAGE

Try to turn undressing into a game in which you can teach some simple concepts and the words for them. For example, some very good concepts and words to work on with undressing are on–off, clothing items, and body parts. So, just before you undress your child, say, "The sock is ON," and then pull off the sock and say, "Now it's OFF! Oh, it's your little foot—I love your little foot!" And then swoop in for kisses or tickles to the foot to keep the activity fun. Before you take off your child's shirt, say, "Shirt is ON," then take off her shirt and say, "Shirt is OFF! Oh, it's your little belly—I love your little belly!" and aim the kisses, tickles, and raspberries to the belly. You can do the same routine for any article of clothing you remove. If your child is starting to say words, you can do this until she is familiar with the routine, and then when you take the shirt off, say "Now shirt is . . ." And pause for her to say "off." If she doesn't say it, you complete it for her: "Shirt is off!"

8. WHERE DID BABY GO?   SOCIAL ENGAGEMENT/LANGUAGE/THINKING

Dressing is a great time to teach the words for body parts as well as the idea that when something is hidden it still exists and that simple interactions with adults can be fun. As you change the child into new clothes, make it a hiding game. For example, you could say, "Here come the PJs over baby's head!" Then as you put the pajamas over his head and can't see him, you could say, "Oh no! Where did baby go?" Then as you pull his head through, say "There he is! There's my baby! Uh-oh! Where is baby's arm? Where did it go?" (the more you can ham it up and really seem astonished or baffled, the better) and then, as you pull his first arm through, say, "Oh, there it is! There is baby's arm!" and so on. If your child is still interested once he's dressed, try to stretch it out even more by hiding Mommy or dolly behind a piece of clothing or a towel. If he takes the initiative to hide or cover his face, you can begin a full-on hunt: "Where did my baby go? He was here just a minute ago! But now I cannot find him anywhere! Is he behind the curtain? NO. Is he under the crib? NO. Is he in the drawer? NO. Oh, there you are! There's my baby!" Your enthusiasm and joy when you find him will reinforce the game and keep the fun going.

 9. GETTING THE PANTS   LANGUAGE/THINKING

Lay out the child's clothes on the bed or floor. You stand a few feet away from her. Say, "Go and get me the socks," or "Get the socks," or even just "Socks," while holding out your hand. If the child gets the socks and gives them to you (or even just one sock), give her praise and a tickle or swing her around—anything she likes. If she doesn't understand the words, hold up a picture of a sock so she can match it to the sock on the bed or floor. Try this with a standard black-and-white line drawing. If this routine becomes easy for your child, you can raise the difficulty level by getting one sock and placing the other on the bed with another very different-looking piece of clothing (for example, a yellow sock and a red sweatshirt). Ask your child, "Can you find the MATCH?" or "Can you find SAME?" As she gets better at this you can gradually put harder choices on the bed, such as other socks that look similar to the sock you want her to get.

Using a Photo of the Child's Clothing

If she doesn't understand matching the real sock to the black-and-white picture, try it with a photograph of her actual sock. Prompt as necessary; for example, you can give her the picture and help her put it on the item of clothing and say, "Look! It's the same" or "Yes! It matches!" You can even do that and then put the sock in her hand and help her hand it to you and then praise her enthusiastically. Remember—praise and reinforce the desired behavior, even if the child needed lots of prompting to be successful.

Using Dressing Puzzles

There are lots of dressing puzzles you can buy; if you have one, you can remove the puzzle pieces that correspond to the articles of clothing in which you're going to dress your child. Then you can help the child put in each puzzle piece as you put the corresponding article of clothing on her; for example, you put her shirt on, then hand her the puzzle piece of the shirt and let her put it in (or help her put it in, if she needs help). When she's done with dressing, the puzzle is done. Similarly, if you have a book about dressing (for example, *Jesse Bear, What Will You Wear?* by Nancy White Carlstrom, or *Blue Hat, Green Hat* by Sandra Boynton), you can alternate between looking at and reading the page about putting on pants and dressing your child in real life (putting on the child's pants).

 10. MOMMY'S SHIRT, BABY'S SHIRT   LANGUAGE/IMITATION/THINKING

Lay out one of your shirts and one of the child's shirts on a bed, low table, or the floor. Ask the child to pick up "Mommy's shirt" or "baby's shirt." Give him as much help as he needs. Then reinforce this in whatever way is fun for him—it could be tossing the shirt up in the air, covering his head with it and then pulling it off, or covering your own head with it and pulling it off—while praising him for picking the right shirt, even if he needed help. If a tickle while you're praising him is something he likes, do that. A good prompt would be to point to the shirt you want him to pick up. For some children, it helps if you point to it while you are very close, or even touching the shirt with your pointer finger. If he needs it, actually hold his hand to pick up the right shirt. The smallest prompt is pointing from a distance, a stronger prompt is prompting from very close, and the strongest prompt involves hand-over-hand help (see the box below). You could also try putting the correct

---

HAND-OVER-HAND HELP

Occasionally, children get upset when you try to give them hand-over-hand help. If that happens, back off and try the other kinds of prompts we describe. But don't necessarily give up on hand-over-hand prompting, because there may be times when that is the only method you can use that will guarantee your child's success with a certain skill and you want to be sure he has plenty of opportunities to be reinforced for practicing new skills correctly. To work your way slowly back to hand-over-hand prompting, try just a brief, gentle touch on the hand or arm to direct the child to pick up the right object, releasing your hand before your child has an opportunity to become upset. Increase the time you keep your hand on your child's hand or arm only very gradually, over a period of days, weeks, or even months. Follow your child's lead and go as slowly as you need to in order to keep things positive!

shirt very close to him and the other one farther away so it's easier (or more likely) for him to choose the correct one. In any case, remember to fade your prompts gradually over time until your child can follow your instructions independently. So, for example, if you used a point to prompt your child, fade your prompt by pointing from farther and farther away and then try just looking in the direction of the shirt you've asked him to get. Eventually you'll want to eliminate your help altogether, so that your child is choosing the shirt you've asked for without any help or hints at all.

Next Steps: "My" and "Your"

If your child is consistently choosing the correct shirt, try teaching him the words "my" and "your" instead of using names. You can prompt by pointing to him when you say "you" and placing an open palm against your own chest as you say the word "my." You can also use "my turn" and "your turn" as you put a little lotion on the baby and then a little lotion on you, or wash baby's face and then wash Mommy's face.

Colors and Sizes

You can also work on colors ("Give me the [pause] BLUE one!"), or you could work on size ("Give me the [pause] LITTLE one!").

11. SILLY DRESSING   SOCIAL ENGAGEMENT/THINKING

If your child knows where the different articles of clothing go (pants on legs, socks on feet, etc.), you can try doing something very silly to see if she finds it funny. For example, while dressing her, you could put on her pants and then her shirt while saying, "The pants go on the legs," and then, "The arms go through the sleeves; the shirt comes down over the belly." Then do something silly, like putting her socks on her hands while saying, "The socks go on the hands—OOPS! Silly! Let's try that again. The sock goes on the foot! The other sock goes on the ear. OOPS! Silly!"—to try to get the child to laugh and perhaps eventually correct your behavior by putting the clothing in the right place. You could also try being silly by putting her clothing on you. For example, "Mommy's shirt goes on Mommy. Just right. Baby's shirt goes on Baby. Just right. Baby's sock goes on Mommy [maybe it just fits over your toe]. OOPS! Too little! That's so silly! Baby's sock goes on Baby. Just right." Don't hesitate to be silly—once children understand the right way to do something, they find it very funny when you deliberately do it the wrong way. Just be sure to then correct it so they get to see it done the right way—the way they expect.

CHAPTER 7

Mealtime

Mealtime is an especially great time to work on teaching your child to request things and make choices. After all, when a child is ready for a snack or meal, food will be a powerful reward. Having a good appetite is a good thing, of course, but if your child is very hungry when mealtime starts, she may get extremely frustrated if you try to work on requesting or making choices. If you think she is feeling very hungry, it might be a good idea to give her some of her food as you usually do, just to take the edge off the child's hunger before you start to work on requesting or making choices.

 ## 1. MORE CHEESE, PLEASE NONVERBAL COMMUNICATION/EYE CONTACT

When you sit down to a meal or snack, try giving your child only a small amount of his favorite food, less than usual, and place a bowl with more of the same food where he can clearly see it. When he finishes with the food on his plate or in his bowl, wait to see if he points to the bowl with more of the food. If he doesn't, you might move it a little closer to him and, if necessary, prompt him to point at it by gently taking his index finger and helping him point to or even touch the bowl before putting more of the food in his plate. Try to get at least a second or two of eye contact just before or after you help him point. If necessary, make it easy for him to make eye contact with you by holding the bowl of food just below your face momentarily where he will naturally see you when he looks at it.

74

More Juice, Please

You can do the same thing with drinks. For example, pour the child only a tiny amount of juice instead of a whole cup. When he finishes that, he'll likely want more. Put the container of juice where he can see it and help him point to it by gently taking his index finger and pointing it toward the juice or even touching the juice container. You can say, "Oh, you want more juice. Here you go!" You can repeat this a few times, helping him point to what he wants, rewarding him right away with more food or more juice, and not making him wait, to prevent him from getting frustrated.

Adding a Word

If your child is learning to say some words, see if you can get him to add a word or a sound to his request. So, for example, if he has been requesting waffles and seems eager for more, try prompting him to say "waffles" or even just the "w" sound. And, of course, make sure that when he requests his food, either by looking at you and pointing to the food he wants or by adding a sound or a word, you give it to him immediately and let him know how happy you are that he did such a nice job asking.

Don't Practice for Too Long at a Time

Remember, though, if any of this seems to be difficult for your child and he seems to become frustrated when you're working on requesting during mealtimes, you should practice it only two or three times during a single meal. Just put more of the food on his plate each time he makes a request. There will be plenty of opportunities to practice this skill with your child, since he eats several times a day, and you can build in more practice at each meal over time. You don't want to frustrate your child or make mealtimes unpleasant, and making sure he gets his basic nutrition should always come first.

2. GRAPES OR BLUEBERRIES?   NONVERBAL COMMUNICATION

Mealtime also provides the perfect opportunity to offer your child choices. Offering either a bite of food or a sip of a drink, or one kind of food or another, is a great way to work on making choices. Simply hold up both choices, such as a grape and a blueberry, or a piece of cheese and a piece of turkey, in front of your child and look at her expectantly. You can ask, "Which one?" or "Which one would you like now?" some of the time, but it's best not to ask every time. Instead, once she has the idea, just hold up the two choices and let your child initiate making a choice. If she doesn't make a choice, prompt her to point to whichever one you think she might like to have. For example, if she has been eating bites of chicken, perhaps she would like a sip of her milk. In that case, just put down the other choice and prompt her to point to the cup. Then say, "Milk" or "Baby wants milk!" and give her a sip right away. As before, try to get a second or two of eye contact before you give her what she chose, but don't wait too long.

 ## 3. USING PICTURES TO REQUEST

If your child is not yet ready to learn to use his words to make requests, try pictures. You might start with clipping pictures of two foods that your child likes to eat from a magazine or printing pictures you download from the Internet. To make them last longer, cover them with a sticky transparent plastic sheet of paper that you can get at a stationery or office supply store. Many stores sell packages of self-laminating sheets that are easy to use and don't require a laminating machine. The pictures should be two or three inches on a side so the child can handle them easily. Make sure you have both foods available, and then put the two pictures on the tray of your child's high chair or on the table if he sits at the table. Whichever one he points to, touches, or hands to you is the one he gets. You can give him just a spoonful or a few small pieces of finger food. If he does not point to one of the pictures or pick one up, you can prompt him by gently placing one of your hands over his and helping him pick up the picture and put it into your other, outstretched hand. Then give him the food he has 'asked for' (even if he doesn't yet understand that he has asked for it).

Work on Eye Contact

You can also use the opportunity to work on eye contact. After your child has touched, pointed to, or handed you a picture, and hasn't made eye contact with you, prompt him to make eye contact (briefly is okay) by holding the food or spoon near your eyes before you give it to him. If he doesn't make eye contact within a few seconds, bring the piece of food 8 to 12 inches in front of his eyes, in the direction of his gaze, so that he will surely see it and then move it toward your own eyes so that he can track it. As soon as he makes eye contact, give him the food. You can do that a few times, but if he is getting frustrated, go back to just working on the point or the picture exchange for a while. After he seems to be getting the idea of making a choice, you can introduce a few new pictures, just presenting two at a time and always making sure you have these foods readily available so you can reward him for requesting by immediately giving him what he has requested.

 ## 4. PICTURE MENU

Once your child can make a choice between two pictures to request a specific food or drink, you can make up a little baby menu with pictures of different favorite foods that are always available (like toast or Cheerios or cheese) and ask your child what she would like to eat. An example is shown on page 77. If you laminate the pictures individually, you can attach them to the menu with Velcro, making it easy

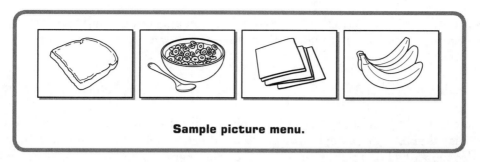

Sample picture menu.

to change the pictures that show her what's available for the meal you are feeding her. It's best not to offer exactly the same choices at every meal or every day, so even if your child has certain favorites that you would like to offer all or most of the time, be sure to offer a variety of different foods, depending on what you happen to have available that day, and change the pictures from meal to meal or day to day. Don't put more than six or so pictures on the page at any one meal. Also, if you notice that your child tends to choose only one or two foods, try leaving that choice off now and then, replacing it with other things you know she enjoys, to encourage her to make some different choices. Show your child the pictures to encourage pointing and making choices. If she doesn't indicate a preference, point to the pictures one by one and show her what you have. For example, at breakfast you might say, "We have oatmeal, peaches, toast, pancakes, and eggs. How about an egg?" Then point to the picture of the egg, or if you have already prepared an egg, remove the picture from the menu and hold it up next to a spoonful of egg and again and say, "Egg," then point to your child and say, "For Baby." Repeat this a couple of times, pointing in turn to the egg and to your child, saying, "An egg for Baby" each time. (Of course, you will substitute your child's name for "Baby.")

 ## 5. HERE COMES THE SPOON! EYE CONTACT

If you're still feeding your child at least some of the time, it's especially easy to work on eye contact during mealtimes by requiring eye contact for each spoonful or piece of food that you offer. Simply hold up a spoonful or a piece of food, and as soon as your child makes eye contact with you, give him a big smile while putting the food into his mouth. When necessary, prompt eye contact by holding the spoon very close to your eyes. For some children, eye contact is difficult, so be satisfied with very brief eye contact (less than 1 second), at least to start with. As it gets easier, you can require a bit longer eye contact, but not more than 2 or 3 seconds (time it—it's longer than you think!). Another way to prompt eye contact is to pretend the spoon is a toy vehicle, like a train or a plane, and fly it around in the air while making engine sounds. When your child is paying attention, pause the spoon near your eyes. As soon as your child makes even brief eye contact with you, offer him a bite while praising him ("Nice looking!"). If your child is partial to vehicles, you can do the same thing with toys when he is finished eating. For example, you can make a toy airplane fly around the room, bring it near your eyes to get eye contact, and then either give him the toy to play with or make it fly again—whichever you think he wants.

6. SILLY MOMMY!   NONVERBAL COMMUNICATION/LANGUAGE

One way to get your child problem solving, and ideally communicating with you, is to "play dumb." For example, you could hand her a cookie that you've put inside a sealed zipper bag or a tightly sealed plastic container or an unopened juice box with the straw removed. The important thing is that the child clearly sees that something she wants is inside a container that she will need your help to open. Then wait for her to communicate in some way that she needs help. She should look at you with a questioning or confused look or perhaps hold the container up to you as a way of asking for your help.

Whatever she does, immediately reinforce her attempts at communication by helping her open the container and giving it back to her. As you do so, you can say something like, "Silly Mommy! It's in a bag! I'll help!" Or, "Silly Mommy! No straw! I'll help!" We hope these situations will encourage your child to look at your face and try to problem-solve how to let you know what she wants.

If you do this once or twice each day with a variety of different things, you can begin to work on getting your child to do just a bit more to get your help. For example, if your child simply looks at you, you could prompt her to lift the container toward you. But if she's already doing that, you could prompt her to say or sign the word "help" or the word "open."

If she is not yet speaking or able to imitate sounds and words, and is not initiating any attempt to get your help, you can prompt the child physically to make the sign for "help" (see the drawing below; Chapter 17 includes pictures of some other useful basic signs).

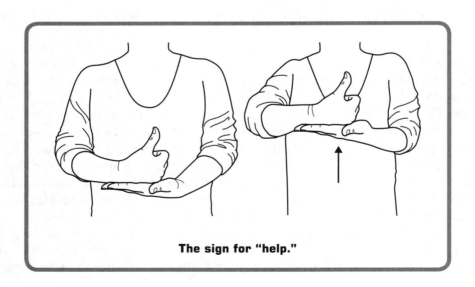

The sign for "help."

Make Your Sentences More Complex

A good way to encourage language development is to use sentences that are just a little more complex than the ones your child is using, about half of the time that you're speaking to her. For example, if your child isn't talking, make sure there are plenty of times during the day that you're using only one word at a time to communicate. In this case, you might just use the word "help" or "open." If your child is using one word at a time, try using sentences with an extra word or two. For example, if your child says "juice," you could respond by pairing the word "juice" with just one other word, like "apple juice," "open juice," "Baby's juice," or "drink juice." The rest of the time, just talk to her naturally, but still try to keep it simple.

Prompt Your Child to Make Her Communication More Complex

In addition, you can prompt the child to add a word to her communication attempt. You shouldn't do this *every* time, because you don't want her to become frustrated, but maybe every other time or every third time you could prompt for just a little bit more before you jump in and help. So, for example, if your child hands you the sealed juice box without a straw, and says, "Juice?" you could prompt her to say, "Open juice?" or "Help juice?" or "Juice straw?"

7. HOT AND COLD   LANGUAGE

If you're about to serve something to your child and you think it's too warm for him to put into his mouth, let him touch it with a finger while you say "hot" and then take it back and blow on it. To teach the difference between hot and cold, you could let the child touch the hot food (not too hot, of course) while you say "hot," then give him an ice cube to touch and say "cold." After doing this a few times, you can try the filling-in procedure where you leave things out, saying, "This one is hot and this one is _____." Try prompting with "c" or "co" if needed. If your child doesn't fill in "cold," finish the sentence for him.

8. "CUT," "BIG," AND "LITTLE"   LANGUAGE

Teaching "Cut"

You can use a knife and say "cut" each time you cut a piece of food in front of your child. For example, if your child likes bananas, peel a banana and put the peeled banana on a plate just out of your child's reach. Put an empty plate in front of her. Cut her one slice of banana at a time and place it on her plate. Each time you cut a piece of the banana, say "cut." Wait for her to eat her slice of banana before you cut the next slice.

After you've cut a few pieces, if your child can imitate the word "cut," or even the "c" sound, hold the knife just above the banana and look at your child with an expectant look. If she says "cut" or "c" or even "banana" or "b," immediately cut her another slice of banana while smiling and saying, "Cut banana!" in a happy tone of voice. If she doesn't say anything when you pause with the knife held just above the banana, prompt her to say what you think she can say and then proceed as if she had done so on her own. If she cannot say "cut" or "c," keep going with the routine, because just being exposed to simple language in a context that makes its meaning clear will be helpful.

Teaching "Big" and "Little"

You can also work on teaching the concept of big and little by making the pieces different sizes. Hold up two pieces and say, "Big piece or little piece?" Wait to see if your child will point to one of the pieces or use one of the words. If so, give her what she asked for and say, "Oh, you want the *big* piece—here you go!" Or, "Oh, you chose the *little* piece." If she doesn't point to one of them, but reaches for one, put the other one down and gently form her hand into a point so that she is pointing to the one she reached for. Then give it to her just as if she had pointed to it by herself.

If your child is able to imitate sounds and words, you can prompt her to say "big" or "little," depending on which piece she is reaching for or pointing to. This is a way to gently push her to use more advanced communication skills. **But remember, don't do this *every* time, just *some* of the time. You want to help your child learn better communication skills, but you don't want her to become frustrated or to get discouraged, and it's really, really important that you sometimes reinforce her efforts at communication right away without asking for more, even if you're pretty sure she can do more.** So even if she can imitate or say words, sometimes just give her what she points to, without requiring that she also use her words.

 ## 9. COUNTING WITH FOOD   LANGUAGE

You can offer a few pieces of food at a time and count them as you put them onto your child's plate. For example, if your child likes waffles, cut a waffle into small pieces. Then put two pieces in one hand and hold it out to your child. Say, "Two," or "Two waffle pieces," and then move them onto his plate one at a time with your other hand, counting as you do so: "One, two." If you do this several times a week, counting out only two to five pieces each time, your child might become familiar enough with these number words to begin trying to say them himself. If he can imitate some sounds or words, try using the filling-in procedure to get him to fill in the last number word. For example, if you have three pieces, count, "One, two," and then pause and wait for him to say "three" before you give him the pieces. If he doesn't, fill in "three!" yourself and then give him the pieces. Pause for long enough (about 5 seconds) that he will want to try to say it himself for the reward of getting the bites of food a little more quickly.

10. TEACHING COLOR WORDS   LANGUAGE

If you're trying to teach your child words for colors, you might try making bowls of different-colored Jell-O (you can start with just two primary colors, like red and green or yellow). Put a few spoonfuls of each in separate small bowls. If your child can say words, ask her which one she wants. If she points or reaches to the bowl with the red Jell-O, model saying "red" for her. If she says "red," immediately give her a spoonful of the red Jell-O. If she cannot say "red," you can say, "Which one is red?" If necessary, help her point to the red one and then immediately give her a bite of the red Jell-O. You can use any two foods that are two different colors, but Jell-O is a nice food to use, because the red Jell-O is very red, the green Jell-O is very green, and the yellow Jell-O is very yellow!

 ## 11. VERBAL IMITATION IN THE KITCHEN   LANGUAGE/IMITATION

If your child is not yet speaking or imitating sounds and words, you can use common kitchen items to work on imitation. Once your child starts to babble (that is, make sounds that are like words but aren't real words), you can encourage him to imitate your babbling by doing it into an empty coffee can or paper towel holder or plastic container or anything that creates an interesting echo. Of course, there are also commercially available toy microphones that operate on this idea, and if you have one, you can take turns making babbling sounds into the little toy microphone. If your child enjoys it, it might even keep him busy for a few extra minutes while you set or clear the table. You can encourage him to really imitate your babbling by keeping it simple, like "ba-ba-ba" or "ga-ga-ga," but you should praise any attempt to imitate your babbling, even if it's not accurate. Some children also enjoy hearing their own voices, and so recording the child's babbling and playing it back to him may encourage him to make more sounds.

 ## 12. HIDE AND SEEK IN THE RICE   LANGUAGE/THINKING

A bowl of uncooked rice (or dried lentils or beans) is a fun way to work on the idea of what we call object permanence, which means understanding that if something leaves your sight it still exists. At the same time, you can work on the concept of "where" by hiding an action figure or small toy in the rice and then saying, "Where did it go?" When your child digs the hidden object out of the rice, be very enthusiastic: "YAY! You found it! Let's hide it again. Where did it go?" **Of course, if your child is still at the stage of putting everything in her mouth, be careful not to let her eat any of the uncooked rice or put the small toy or object in her mouth.**

13. FITS OR DOESN'T FIT   LANGUAGE/THINKING

A fun game for toddlers is to see what fits into something else. Try playing this game when your child is sitting at the kitchen table. Try to see what fits into an empty orange juice container, an empty food storage container, through a paper towel roll, into a hole you cut in a shoe box, and so on. Just get your container and a variety of objects that are too big for the child to choke on. Collect objects that either will or will not fit into the container's opening. Hand your child the objects, one by one, and say, "Can you put it *in*?" or even just "*In*?" Give your child whatever help he needs to try to put the objects in the container. If they go in, say, "It's *in*! It *fits*!" And if it doesn't go in, you can say something like "Oops! *Too big*." If your child has more language, you can expand on this by using the names of the objects you've collected. So, for example, if you're using a small plastic zebra figure that's too big to fit through the container's hole, you could say, "Can you put the zebra in?" Then, when it doesn't fit, you could say, "Oops! Zebra is too big! He doesn't fit."

 14. PRETENDING TO FEED DOLLY   PRETEND PLAY/IMITATION

When you are first introducing pretend play, feeding is a great thing to pretend with a favorite doll or stuffed animal, because it's something that your child will be very familiar with. You can bring a doll or a teddy bear to the table or his high chair when your child is finishing his dinner and make baby crying noises and pretend that the baby is hungry. Then use a child's spoon and bowl or a toy bottle and say something like, "Oh, no. Baby's hungry. Let's feed the baby!" Then help the child feed the baby (or the teddy) by gently helping her hold the bottle or spoon and bring it to the baby doll's mouth, then say something like, "Yum. Baby loves the food [or the milk]. Thank you!"

Your child might think it's fun to feed Mommy too. You can lean forward and open your mouth and say, "Feed Mommy?" If she does it, say, "Thank you for sharing! Mommy is so happy!" or just "Thank you." As with all activities, give the child just as much help as she needs and then try to fade your help. So you might have to start by hand-over-hand prompting her to feed you, then it might work to just hand her the spoon with a small bit of food and lean in very close with your mouth open, then she might be able to feed you without your leaning in too far. Then always praise the child, no matter how much help she needed. If she's ready, you could also turn this into a game where you take turns feeding each other.

 15. PRETENDING TO COOK   PRETEND PLAY/IMITATION/LANGUAGE

When you're working in the kitchen, if possible, let your child play near you, with his own little pot and spoon, so he can pretend to do what you're doing. This will help him get the idea that pretend play starts by imitating adult actions. You can also work on language, by labeling his actions, like "Mix, mix" as he stirs his pot, or labeling and demonstrating "fast" and "slow" as you mix with him or show him how to bang the spoon on the pot fast or slow. Anytime you say "fast" or "slow" or "mix" and he does what you say, make a big fuss: "THAT's going fast—what a good drummer!"

If your child can imitate some sequences of things you do, you can set up some toy pots and pans in the kitchen so that your child can "cook" while Mommy or Daddy cooks. If you don't have toy pots, pans, or cooking utensils, just use one or two of your smaller pots and pans and a wooden spoon. Help your child stir the imaginary food in his pot while you stir the real food. Pretend to taste his delicious cooking and offer him a taste of yours. Ask him what he will add next. For example, if you're making a stew, have him pretend to add carrots and potatoes to his pot while you add them to yours. If he has difficulty pretending these things, try using toy food or small pieces of real food to put into his pot. Of course, there are also commercially available toy kitchens with all sorts of pots, pans, dishes, utensils, and foods. If you happen to have one of these, the real kitchen is a great place to keep it if you can make room for it there. But a small, old pot and wooden spoon work very well, too. At first, you may need to do a lot of prompting and reinforcing of your child's pretend cooking. Your pretending to eat his food and finding it delicious may be the biggest reinforcer of all. And if your child begins to enjoy pretending to cook while you cook, his play will keep him busy right nearby for a while so that you can get a meal prepared.

 ## 16. YUMMY/YUCKY FOOD **LANGUAGE/THINKING**

If you're working on what to put in your mouth and what not to, read the book *Yummy Yucky* by Leslie Patricelli and then have Cookie Monster or another stuffed animal or puppet go around the kitchen tasting things that are food and not food and making a big deal out of how delicious the food is and how "yucky" the non-food items are. Use simple phrases that you can repeat over and over. For example, you might say only the words "yummy" and "yucky" using your pretend Cookie Monster voice, and then you can add more words in your own voice, like, "Oh, Cookie Monster! You don't eat napkins! Napkins are yucky!" and "Yay! Good eating apples, Cookie Monster! Apples are yummy!" If your child is paying attention to this game and seems to enjoy it, and can say or imitate a few words, you can go back to some "yummy" and "yucky" items that you've already talked about a few times and ask your child to fill in the right word (for example, "Good eating cheese, Cookie Monster [or other doll or figure]! Cheese is . . .") and then pause for your child to say "yummy." If she doesn't say it, you can prompt her by saying "yummy," and if she imitates you, give her enthusiastic praise ("Good talking!") and a piece of cheese if she likes it.

17. YUMMY AND YUCKY TOOTHPASTE   LANGUAGE

You can continue the yummy and yucky theme when you brush your child's teeth. There are many different flavors of toothpaste on the market—try buying several flavors and colors and using your child's face as a guide to whether you should label it as "yummy" or "yucky." If you get a strong reaction from your child, expand on it even further by showing him his face in the mirror and saying, "You love strawberry! Mmm, mmm delicious!" or "You do not like this toothpaste. Yucky."

 ## 18. GETTING READY FOR TOOTH BRUSHING   LANGUAGE/IMITATION

Instead of getting everything ready for your child before brushing her teeth, involve her by saying, "Squeeze" or "Squeeze the toothpaste," and then use a physical prompt to help her gently squeeze some toothpaste onto her toothbrush. Seeing the toothpaste come out of the tube may be rewarding enough for your child, especially if she likes the toothpaste flavor, but a little extra praise, like, "Wow! Good squeezing!" might be helpful.

You can work on the phrase "turn on" by having your child stand on a stool and gently demonstrating and then prompting her to turn on the cold water when you say, "Turn on." Be sure to emphasize the word "on." (Of course, you want to be careful that she doesn't turn on the hot water!) Water is often a big reward by itself, but again, praise her for doing as you've asked, even if you had to help. Then say, "Turn off," emphasizing the word "off," and prompt your child to turn the water off, followed by more praise. You can do this several times in a row and make a game of it, fading your prompts gradually over several trials. And you can do this at the kitchen sink when you have to fill up a large pot for cooking.

If your child resists having his teeth brushed, it may help to make it a predictable routine: For example, count out the same number of brush strokes each time so that he knows what to expect; be silly (encourage him to brush fast enough to "make foam," make silly faces in the mirror, laugh when you "spit" at the same time); and sing a short tooth-brushing song to him while you're brushing his teeth, trying to end the brushing when the song ends every time you brush. Raffi and Barney both have good tooth-brushing songs, and there are dozens of others on YouTube. Of course, you can always make up your own silly tooth-brushing song too.

 ## 19. BRUSHING DOLLY'S TEETH   IMITATION/PRETEND PLAY

Tooth brushing is another good thing to pretend with a favorite doll or stuffed animal. Just take a doll into the bathroom and, after you finish brushing your child's teeth, take an old toothbrush and say, "Let's brush dolly's teeth," and then help him hold the toothbrush and brush the doll's teeth. If you brush your child's teeth two times every day, this will be another nice, simple routine that he is very familiar with, and it may help him understand the idea of pretending. Keep it simple—just brush the doll's teeth, but if your child seems very interested, you can act out a little more of the tooth-brushing routine, by telling him "water on," getting the brush just a little bit wet, brushing the doll's teeth, and then having the doll bend over the sink and spit ("poo, poo, poo").

 ## 20. FUN WITH FOOD   BEHAVIOR, PRETEND, THINKING, IMITATION

If your child is a very picky eater and you want her to get used to being around foods that smell different or that she doesn't like to eat, try doing some art projects with a little bit of food. The idea is not to encourage the child to eat foods she really dislikes, just to get her used to the sight, smell, and feel of less familiar foods, so don't ask her to eat them. This will mean using only small bits of food that you don't mind wasting. There are many books that show wonderful ideas for art food projects, like *Funny Food* and *Snacktivities*. Or just make up your own, like a marshmallow man with raisins. If she wants to eat your creation, that's fine, but don't require it. You can do this while she's in her high chair before mealtime, and if she doesn't want to eat it, let her feed it to you. That still promotes social interaction and gives you a chance to praise her for feeding you.

CHAPTER 8

Bathtime

Bathtime is another great time to work on the words for body parts as well as the concepts of wet and dry and action words like "splash," "jump," "pour," "wash," and "rinse." There are other concepts too, like full and empty, or sticks and doesn't stick. Here are some ideas for how to work on these things while giving your child a bath.

 ## 1. WET AND DRY, HEAD AND TUMMY   LANGUAGE

As you first put your baby in the bath, most of his body will be dry. Use simple, repetitive phrases to teach the concepts of wet and dry and to work on words for parts of the body. For example, say, "Now Baby's tummy is dry." (You can use the child's name instead of "Baby.") Then pour some water onto his tummy and say, "Now, Baby's tummy is wet!" And then: "Now Baby's arm is dry." "Now Baby's arm is wet." "Now Baby's shoulder is dry." "Now Baby's shoulder is wet." After you've done this routine several times, try using the filling-in procedure to see if your child will fill in the words ("Baby's nose is *dry*." Put a drop of water on his nose and say "Now Baby's nose is . . ."). If he doesn't try to fill it in, say it for him. If he tries to say "wet," be enthusiastic: "Yes! Baby's nose is *wet*." Having the warm water wash over his body should feel nice to him. If so, pouring the water may be a great natural reinforcer for saying the body part word because he'll know that the next pour of water is coming.

You can use the same phrasing to demonstrate wet and dry with your washcloths and sponges too: "Now the washcloth is dry. Now the washcloth is wet." After doing this a few times, you can try the filling-in procedure, saying, "Sponge

86

is dry. [Dunk the sponge.] Now sponge is wet. Washcloth is dry. [Dunk the washcloth.] Now washcloth is wet. Ring [bathtub rubber toy ring] is dry. [Dunk the ring.] Now ring is . . ." Pause for a few seconds to give your child time. If he doesn't try to say "wet," you say, "Ring is *wet*!" Or you could say, "Ring is w . . . ," using the "w" sound as a prompt, and wait for him to fill it in. If he doesn't, you finish it for him.

 ## 2. I SPLASH, YOU SPLASH   IMITATION

Since splashing is so much fun, it's a good opportunity to practice imitating simple actions. Say, "Do this!" and gently splash some water onto the tub or gently hit the surface of the water. If the child doesn't make an attempt to imitate you, prompt her by taking her hand and imitating your action. Or you can begin by imitating something the child is doing, just to get her attention focused on interaction. Then say, "Do this!" and reinforce her splash even if she needed a hand-over-hand prompt ("That's right! You splashed, too"). If she does make an attempt, praise even more enthusiastically ("That's right! You did what I did"). Then work on making her imitation more precise, by doing different kinds of splashing (splashing the tub wall, gently splashing her tummy, hitting the water, splashing with a small toy, etc.).

If you think she's ready for it, try having her imitate you putting a spot of bubbles on various body parts. Using bubble bath or bath foam, which has the consistency of shaving cream, put a small dot of bubbles on her nose, shoulder, arm, and so on, one body part at a time, and have her imitate you. Put some bubbles on her finger and say, "Now you do it! Put it on your arm." As always, if the child makes no attempt to "do this," prompt and reinforce. If she makes an incorrect attempt, praise her for the attempt and then show her the correct body part with a prompt. ("Good try! Here's your arm. Look! Now you have two bubble circles on your arm.") You can also work on her understanding the correspondence between her body parts and yours, by putting a dab of bubble bath on your nose, cheek, forehead, arm, or fingers and saying, "Now you do it! Put it on yours," and, as always, if she doesn't do it, gently prompt with hand-over-hand guidance and reinforce: "Yes! That's mine, and that's yours!" or "Yes! That's my nose, and that's your nose."

 ## 3. BUBBLES ON BODY PARTS   LANGUAGE

Using bubble bath or bath foam, place little dabs of bubbles or cream on different parts of your face and your child's face, labeling "Mommy's nose, Baby's nose," or "Mommy's cheek, Baby's cheek." You can also offer choices for where to put the bath foam next. For example, you could ask, "Should I put it on your hand or your belly?" while pointing to each in turn. You can use a hand mirror to show her the bubbles on her face. If the child points to the body part, labels it verbally, or lifts it up (like a hand or foot), put the bubbles where he has indicated. Once you have put it on, wipe it off and say, "All gone." This is similar to the game "I Splash, You

Splash," but there you were concentrating on teaching imitation, while here you are concentrating on teaching your child the words for different body parts. Feel free to mix them up, however, and do them together. You're the best judge of how simple to make the games to best engage your child and help him understand more language.

4. MAKING BATHTUB CHOICES   NONVERBAL COMMUNICATION

When you give your child a bath, you may want to try having lots of different textures available, such as a sea sponge, a gauze sponge, a loofah glove, shaving cream or bath foam, bubble bath, and a washcloth. After exposing the child to each, you might try holding up two choices at a time and seeing whether she'll reach for one. If she's reliably able to reach out to make this kind of choice, put down the other one and, with your free hand, try gently shaping her fingers into a point and helping her point to the one she wants, even touching it with the outstretched finger. Then immediately hand her whatever thing she has chosen and use her choices for her bath. You could do this with washcloth versus sponge, then try it with two bath toys, then perhaps with two bath crayons. Remember that you're trying to get across the idea that pointing to something is a way to request it, so try to immediately reinforce this attempt by giving the child or using whatever she has chosen.

5. BATH SONGS   LANGUAGE

As you wash each part of your child's body, sing about it to a familiar tune. For example, you could sing, "This is the way we wash" to the tune of "Here We Go Round the Mulberry Bush." Just sing about whatever body part you're washing. So, for example, when you're washing your child's back, you would sing, "This is the way we wash your back, wash your back, wash your back; this is the way we wash your back when we take a tubby."

Feel free to use whatever song you think your child might like best. For example, you could sing a slightly different song to the tune of "The Wheels on the Bus," which would go like this: "Now I'm washing Baby's feet, Baby's feet, Baby's feet. Now I'm washing Baby's feet. Now his [or her] feet are clean." In any case, you would repeat the verses for rinsing, drying, and rubbing lotion onto each body part, singing "rinsing," "drying," and "rubbing." You can end by offering tickles and kisses for each body part. And once your child becomes familiar with these songs, remember to use the filling-in procedure and see if he'll fill in the blanks.

And there's a great song for washing hair. You could sing, "I'm gonna wash that dirt right out of your hair" to the tune of "I'm Gonna Wash That Man Right Out of My Hair" from *South Pacific* during shampoos (check YouTube if you're not familiar with it). It would go like this: "I'm gonna wash that dirt right out of your hair. I'm gonna wash that dirt right out of your hair. I'm gonna wash that dirt right out of your hair and send it down the drain." As with all the other activities, your child has to be paying attention for these games to be useful. If you can't get his attention and see no evidence of enjoyment, move on to something else.

 ## 6. DOLLY'S BATH PRETEND PLAY/LANGUAGE

If your child is really enjoying these bathtime songs, you can sing the same songs while washing a waterproof doll, animal, or character toy, so that she sees one of her favorite toys getting the same scrub-down she got. And she'll get another chance to hear and perhaps say all those words again. If she's interested, give her the doll and the washcloth or sponge and suggest she wash the dolly's back, arm, hair, and so on, and then prompt her gently: "That's dolly's hair! Let's wash dolly's hair." If she does not independently wash the doll, prompt her by gently helping her hold the washcloth, dunk it, and wash dolly's foot or arm or hair and then praise her ("Yay! You washed dolly's hair!"), and if she likes it, you could gently splash some water on her belly, or anything else she likes in the tub, as a reinforcer. Remember—if your child needs a prompt to do something, you should still reinforce it as if she had done it by herself, giving a little less help each time if she's learning to do it by herself.

 ## 7. SPLASHING HANDS AND FEET LANGUAGE

Try teaching your child to "splash" with his hands and also with his feet. Take his feet and gently kick them against the surface of the water, saying, "Splash with your feet," and then do the same with his hands and say, "Splash with your hands." Next, you can take a bath crayon (these are wonderful things to have) and draw some little people or animals on the side of the tub and show your child how to "splash doggie," "splash bunny," and so on. You can prompt him by physically helping him splash the right drawing (it's easiest to start with just two). As always, even if he needs a prompt, reinforce him with enthusiastic praise as if he had done it himself. When the figures you drew begin to disappear, or you rub them out, say good-bye to the animals in turn—for example, "Goodbye, doggie," "Goodbye, bunny." If you think your child can rub out the drawing, you can say, "Goodbye, bunny," and prompt him to rub out the correct drawing.

 ## 8. JUMP, SPLASH, SQUIRT LANGUAGE

If you have some small tub animals, line them up on the side of the bath and have each one jump into the bath, saying, "Jump, splash!" and then do it again adding the animal names: "Froggy, jump, splash," "Duck, jump, splash." Then if you have a toy that squirts, try, "Froggy, squirt Baby; Froggy, squirt Mommy," and really laugh to let your child know this is a pretty funny game! Anytime you get your child laughing, say "silly" "funny" or "happy" to name the emotion for her.

9. TUB TOY CLEAN-UP

If you have a net or basket for storing bath toys, leave the toys stored when you first put your child in the bath so that you can ask him if you should take them out, one by one. This will give you an opportunity to use a repetitive language approach to work on language. For example, you might ask, "Froggy out?" If your child says yes, or nods his head, or even if he just reaches for the toy, say, "Okay, Froggy out!" and take Froggy out of the storage net or basket with a flourish as you say the word "out." Then ask about the next toy, and so on, until your child has plenty of bath toys in the tub to play with. If you want your child to focus on only one or two toys at a time, line up some of the others around the edge of the tub when you take them out.

Near the end of the bath, try taking turns with your child, putting different bath toys in the net or basket when you say the word "in." You can also name the objects as you store them. For example, you could say, "Froggy in," and make Froggy hop into the net or basket. Then you can say, "Your turn! Ducky in!" If your child makes no move to put the duck in the basket, hand it to him; if he still doesn't put it in, gently help him put it in, then praise him as if he had done it by himself.

 10. STICKS OR DOESN'T STICK

There are lots of foam and plastic letters, numbers, vehicles, and animals that are meant to stick to the side of the tub.

You can try teaching your child to put these up on the wall, saying, "It sticks!" or just "Sticks!" and also mix in some regular bath toys that won't stick. When you put those up, say, "Doesn't stick," or "Oops—it fell down" (and laugh when the toys hit the water—anything you laugh at will hold more interest for your child). If your child enjoys this routine, it can also be played with felt and nonfelt items on a felt board when your child finishes her bath. Your foam tub figures, for example, will probably not stick to the felt board. You can also carry this concept over to the kitchen by handing him small magnetic and nonmagnetic items and see if they stick on the refrigerator, labeling them: "Oh, it sticks!" or "Oops! It doesn't stick."

 11. FLOATS OR SINKS

One way to play "Float or Sink" is to get a bucket of various objects and put them into the tub, one at a time, commenting on whether it "sinks" or "floats." Your child might enjoy it even more if you drop it in from a little way up, make a fuss about the suspense ("Will it sink or float? I don't know") and then, when it pops up or stays down, say, "It sinks!" or "It floats!" Another way to play is to make floating boats out of aluminum foil and then see how many figurines or other toys it takes to sink them.

12. BATHTUB COLORS

LANGUAGE/THINKING

A drop of food coloring or some fizzy colored bath tablets can be really fun in the bath. Take any opportunity you can to let your child make a choice between two colors. Hold up two different colors and then when she reaches for one say, "Oh you want the *red* one." Drop in the tablet or food coloring and give her a big wooden spoon to stir in the color. Then praise her, saying something like, "Wow, you did it! You made it red!" If she likes this, you can find more ways to reinforce the concept of red such as sorting red and non-red bath toys. For example, say, "I'm going to get all of our red bath toys. Here's a red one; it goes in the bath. Here's another red one! It goes in the bath too! Oops, not red. Let's leave it out." When you get out of the bath, see if you can keep it going by drying your child in a red towel and putting her in red PJs.

 ## 13. FILL AND SPILL

THINKING/LANGUAGE

Get some plastic or paper cups and show your child how to "fill . . ." (rising intonation) and "spill" the water (falling intonation) as he sits in the tub. After all, what child doesn't enjoy pouring water? Use a repetitive language approach and the filling-in procedure to teach these two words. Each time you fill a cup with water, say, "First we fill, and then we spill." As you say the word "spill," spill the water out of the cup. After a while, pause before saying the words "fill" and "spill" and see if your child will fill in the blanks. When he does (or tries to say it), cheer for him and hand him another cup of water to pour out! You can do the same thing with "pour" and "more" by saying, "First we pour, and then we get more!"

 ## 14. DRYING OFF SONG

LANGUAGE/SOCIAL ENGAGEMENT

When your child gets out of the bath, wrap her in a fluffy towel (a towel fresh out of the dryer is especially comfy and attention grabbing) and give her a massage with lotion, unless she does not like that. You can sing the washing bath song to the tune of "Here We Go Round the Mulberry Bush," but replace the word "wash" with the word "dry" when you're drying your child with the towel and with the word "rub" when you're putting on her lotion or powder. For example, when you're drying her with the towel you can sing, "This is the way we dry your arms, dry your arms, dry your arms. This is the way we dry your arms, after we take a tubby," and then when you're rubbing the lotion on her, sing, "This is the way we rub your arms, rub your arms, rub your arms. This is the way we rub your arms when we put on lotion."

CHAPTER 9

Chores

Almost any chore can be used to teach more language, as well as imitation and pretend play. Here are some examples. Use your creativity and adapt them to any chore you're doing.

 ## 1. DRIVING TO THE WASHING MACHINE

NONVERBAL COMMUNICATION/ LANGUAGE/PRETEND PLAY

Pretend your laundry basket is a boat or car that your child can "drive." This will work best if you have a wide, shallow laundry basket in which the child can fit comfortably and can see over the sides. You can give her a round toy to use as a wheel and help her "drive" the laundry basket; if necessary, prompt her by holding her hands on the round toy and showing her how to turn the wheel left and right, then praise her (for example, "You're driving! What a good driver! Here we go!").

Teaching "Fast" and "Slow"

You can work on "fast" and "slow" by putting your child on top of the clothes in the laundry basket and pushing the laundry basket to and from the washing machine at different rates and then wait for your child to communicate with you. If you go out of your house or apartment to do laundry, of course you can still let your child "drive" around the house with the laundry basket. You can say, "Fast!" while pushing or pulling the basket fast and then, "Slooooowwww," while pushing it very slowly. Then ask your child if she wants "fast" or "slow." If she can't say these words, you can ask, "Do you want fast?" and help her nod "yes" by demonstrating it yourself.

Teaching "Stop" and "Go"

Then you can do the same thing with "go" and "stop." Stop and go as you move about the house on your way to the washing machine. When you stop, wait for your child to communicate with you before pushing the basket again. If your child is not yet speaking, she may simply rock her body to indicate that she wants you to go, and that's fine—any attempt at communication should be rewarded as long as she is looking at you. You can make it easier for her to look at you by pulling instead of pushing the basket so you're right in front of her. And, of course, if your child loves trains, give her a ride in a laundry basket train with her as the conductor: "Choo-choo! All aboard!"

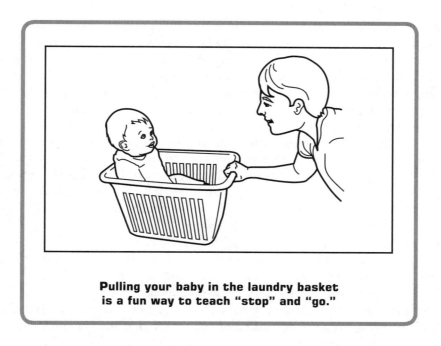

**Pulling your baby in the laundry basket
is a fun way to teach "stop" and "go."**

 ## 2. THE LAUNDRY ROUTINE   EYE CONTACT/NONVERBAL COMMUNICATION

When you're ready to put the clothes into the washing machine, you can have your child hand you the pieces of clothing one at a time, and then you can put them into the machine. Start by holding out your hand and saying, "Give me one." Prompt the child with hand-over-hand help if needed to reach into the basket and hand you a piece of clothing. If your child can reach the opening of the machine, or if there's a safe place for him to sit (like on the dryer or another washing machine if you can hold on to him), you could hand *him* the clothes and have him toss them in, which might be more fun for him. Wait for him to make eye contact with you before passing each item of clothing. If your child enjoys throwing the clothes into the machine, then releasing each item into his hand is a natural reward for eye contact. If he avoids making eye contact with you, you might try getting his attention by shaking the article of clothing, then moving it up to just next to your eyes to see if you can get him to look at you for just a second, and then giving him the clothing to throw into the machine. **Coordinating movements with another person is a very important skill to learn.**

3. LAUNDRY LANGUAGE   LANGUAGE

Having your child help you with the laundry can provide a great way to work on language too. You can work on articles of clothing, colors, family members, and "wet" and "dry." Label each piece of clothing—"shirt," "pants," "socks," and so on—as you hand it to your child to put into the washing machine or dryer. Or, if your child is ready to understand two words, you could label the articles of clothing and add a color word, like "blue shirt" or "white sock." You can even work on the names of family members and the idea of possession by saying whose clothing you're holding as you hand over each piece. For example, you could say, "Mommy's shirt," or "Baby's sock." For an older child with more language, you can ask, "Whose socks are these?" or "What color is this shirt?"

You can do similar routines when putting the wet clothes into the dryer and when folding the clothes once they're dry. You can work on the words "wet" and "dry" by labeling the items as "wet" as you let the child touch each wet piece of clothing before you place it into the dryer and later labeling those pieces of clothing as "dry" when you remove them from the dryer. If your child is starting to talk, you can prompt her to say "wet" or "dry" by saying, "Sock is wet. Shirt is wet. Underwear is wet. Sock is . . . ," and prompt with a "w" sound if necessary. If she cannot yet say any words, it's still very helpful for her to hear these simple words in situations that help make their meaning clear, like touching the wet clothing.

The activities above work on expressive language, but you can also work on receptive language (understanding language). As you take the dirty clothes out of the laundry basket, hold up two different articles of clothing—a shirt and a sock, for example. Say, "Throw the sock in!" or "Which one is the sock?" When your child reaches for or points to the correct item, cheer for her, then hand it to her and let her throw it in. If she reaches for the incorrect item, just hold both items out of her reach and try again, but the second time, prompt by holding the sock a bit closer to her and the shirt a bit farther away. Your child may find that pushing the start button and either feeling the washing machine vibrate or watching the clothes start to spin for a few seconds is a fun, rewarding way to end this activity.

4. LAUNDRY MATCHING   LANGUAGE/THINKING

When you take the laundry out, help your child sort his clothes from the grownups' clothes or try to make "matches" with socks or underwear. This will help him develop the idea of sorting and matching.

Whose Clothes?

For example, put all the clean clothes on a bed that he can see; make a pile of his clothes and others' clothes. After you've put a few items of clothing into these two piles, hand him an article of clothing and ask, "Where does it go?" If he puts it anywhere but on the correct pile, give it back to him and prompt him to put it on the right pile, saying, "Baby's clothes," or "Mommy's clothes."

Matching Types of Clothes

After you have a pile of your child's clothes, you can put a couple of white socks together and a couple of dark socks together and do the same matching game with the rest of the socks, saying, "Where does it go?" or "Let's match." Prompt him to put the socks in the right pile and praise him enthusiastically even if he needed a prompt.

Matching Sizes

You can also work on big and little. For example, take one of your socks and hold it up next to one of his. Say, "This one is big. It's Mommy's sock," and "This one is little. It's Baby's sock." If your child is starting to say words, you can do this a few times and then hold up a big sock and say, "This one is . . ." Prompt if necessary with "b." Then do it with "little." As always, praise him for correct answering, even if a prompt was needed. Speaking is a difficult skill to prompt. You can prompt a word by speaking the word for the child or giving him the first sound, but it's much harder to actually fully prompt your child to say a word than to put something in the right place because with the latter you can physically prompt him by putting your hand over his hand. So if he doesn't say any words for you, try to end the activity on a successful note by holding up a big sock and a little sock and asking, "Which one is little?" or "Which one is Baby's?" (whichever you think is easier for him) and, if needed, prompting him to reach for the correct sock so that you can enthusiastically reinforce his choice—"Great! You picked the little one!"—even if he needed hand-over-hand help to pick it.

 ## 5. WHERE DOES IT GO? **THINKING**

Put a label on your child's clothes drawers with a picture of what goes there—a picture of pants, socks, underwear, shirts, and so on. Then take the clean laundry and hand her an item and ask, "Where does it go?" You'll have to help your child learn to match the real item with the picture on the dresser at first, so you can gently help her put the item next to the picture, reinforce ("Yes! Good matching! That's where pants go!"), and then help her put the item in the correct drawer or shelf. Give her as much help as she needs and then back off, giving less and less help as she learns to match, and be sure to reinforce with enthusiastic praise, even if she needed help. Watch those little fingers in the drawers, too!

6. THE CLEAN-UP SONG   THINKING/BEHAVIOR

Getting children to help with cleaning up can be a real challenge. Start with just one toy that has to go in a basket or on a shelf, with everything else put away. You can sing the clean-up song that is often sung in preschools ("Clean up, clean up, everybody everywhere, clean up, clean up, everybody do their share")—or any of the many clean-up songs on the Internet—whichever one appeals to you. Guide the child gently to pick up the one toy or book and put it where it goes, then give him a lot of praise and move on to a fun activity. Do this with one toy a few times over several days. Then try leaving two toys out, sing the clean-up song, and guide the child to put the two things away, followed by praise and a treat or a fun activity. Your goal is to get the clean-up song to signal time to put toys or materials away, but for very young children this is a boring and unpleasant activity, so don't expect them to put away more than a few things at a time.

 7. CLEAN-UP SORTING   THINKING

After your child can put away two or three things, you can start to work on the idea of sorting. This may be your child's first chance to start learning how to sort things or how to put similar things together. Clean-up time is a great place to work on that skill, especially if you take a little time to organize your child's toys and books beforehand. That way, you can begin by showing your child that everything has a special place or belongs somewhere. For example, if you have an area on a shelf or a small bin to hold your child's books, another container for her puzzles, another for her blocks, another for her balls, and one more for her cars and trains, you can start to show her that books go in one place and balls or blocks go somewhere else. It helps if you can label the bins or boxes by taking a picture of each one, filled with the toys that belong inside, and then attach the pictures to the bins (see the drawing below). If you can, use clear plastic bins so the child can see what goes inside.

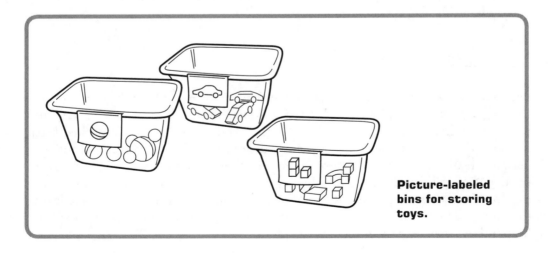

Picture-labeled bins for storing toys.

You can sing the clean-up song and then pick up a ball and say, "It's clean-up time! This is a ball." Then point to your child's bin of balls and say, "Balls go here," and prompt her to put the ball in the bin with the other balls. Then, of course, praise her enthusiastically, give her a tickle or a swing around, or whatever she likes, and show her how happy you are that she is such a big girl cleaning up her toys!

If your child can say some words, you can hold up a toy, such as a puzzle, and ask, "What's this?" If she doesn't answer, you can prompt or answer for her and then ask, "Where do puzzles go?" If she doesn't start toward the right place, guide her gently and point to the place the puzzle belongs, saying, "Puzzles go here! Good cleaning up!" Repeat this process until your child starts to understand what goes where. If it gets boring, it might help to try making a game of it by saying, "Does book go here?" Then put it someplace silly (like on your head) and let your child correct you. Again, don't expect a young child to put away more than four to six objects. This means that before you start to work on cleaning up, it's a good idea to put away everything except four to six things. If the child sees only a few things that need to be put away, she is likely to be less resistant.

 ## 8. SORTING SILVERWARE **THINKING**

If your child is catching on to the idea of sorting, you can have him help when you empty the dishwasher or put away the clean silverware. Seat him at the table or in his high chair and put the empty silverware tray in front of him, next to some of the forks and spoons (no knives!) from the dishwasher baskets or the clean dish basket by the sink. Start by putting a couple of spoons and forks in the right compartments. Then say "Let's match" or "Let's put these away." If he does it correctly, give lots of praise! If he doesn't do it, gently prompt with your hand over his and then praise him. If he does it incorrectly, praise him for a good try and then help him put the forks with the other forks and the spoons with the other spoons ("This is a spoon. Here's where the spoons go"). And if he does it by himself and makes a few mistakes, it's still a good activity for working on fine-motor coordination.

 ## 9. WASHING THE TABLE **IMITATION**

If there is a surface that you can wipe down with just water, this is a good chance to have your child imitate you. She can wipe down her high chair tray or a low table or even a kitchen table if she can reach it while sitting in a chair. You wipe a small section of the table or high chair tray, then hand her a wet sponge or paper towel and say, "You wipe, too!" Prompt if necessary using your hand over hers and helping her wipe the table. Then see if she will do a little piece of it by herself. Praise her enthusiastically for being such a good helper, even if she needed a prompt. Don't worry about anything actually getting clean; you can go over it later. The point here is to teach her to imitate your actions. If you're in the kitchen, you can say something like, "Now we got the table clean, so we can have a tiny snack," and put a small treat for each of you on the "clean" table (like a sweet piece of cereal for each of you). You're teaching your child that food goes on a clean table and providing a reward for imitating you and helping you. (Washing and drying provides another opportunity to practice the concepts of "wet" and "dry" as well as "dirty" and "clean.")

 ## 10. SWEEP, SWEEP, SWEEP!   IMITATION

Sweeping is another good activity for working on imitation. This is best done after you've done the real sweeping, and then you can sprinkle some small pieces of paper towel or something else that will show up against your floor. Don't use anything edible, and watch your child to make sure he doesn't put the pieces in his mouth. Get your child a toy broom or just a small brush that he can handle easily. Sweep a little part of the floor and say, "You help, too," and hand him his brush. Help him sweep the bits into a dustpan and then praise him for being such a good helper.

CHAPTER 10

Errands

Working on skills and using teaching opportunities can be quite a challenge when you're trying to run errands outside of the house with a young child (or more than one). But there are still lots of opportunities for fun games that will teach skills. Some of the activities we describe in this chapter are designed for when you're actually running your errands, and some are designed to be done at home before you leave or after you return. And remember, running errands provides lots of opportunities to work on greeting familiar people and to practice waving bye-bye. Read them through and see what you think will work for you.

 1. WAVING BYE-BYE   NONVERBAL COMMUNICATION/EYE CONTACT/IMITATION

You can work on waving bye-bye either when you and the child are leaving the house or when someone else is leaving. We went through how to teach waving in some detail in Chapter 2. Briefly, when you're leaving the house with the child and there's another adult staying home, or when another adult is leaving the house, ask the other adult to wave and say "bye-bye" to the child. Help the child make eye contact by having the adult who is waving put his face at the child's eye level and wave his hand near his face to draw the child's attention if necessary. If the child does not make any attempt to wave, prompt him gently by raising his hand and moving it back and forth in a waving gesture. Then let go of his hand and praise enthusiastically ("Good waving bye-bye to Susie!"). If the child avoids making eye contact with the adult, just reinforce the waving anyway and look for other opportunities to make eye contact with the child, giving him praise and, if possible, a reward when he does.

99

2. SONGS IN THE CAR

It can be challenging to hold your child's attention while you're in the car or on a bus or train. For a child who is beginning to experiment with sounds and words, you can try singing her favorite songs or saying favorite nursery rhymes, then pausing and seeing if she'll try to say the next word in the song or nursery rhyme. For example, if you sing the Winnie the Pooh song over and over, eventually you can begin with "Winnie the _____," and pause before you say "Pooh." Or if you sing "The Itsy Bitsy Spider," you can pause before important words, like "spider," "sun," and "rain." This technique of leaving out a word or a sound and seeing if the child will fill it in is useful in figuring out how much your child knows, and also at keeping her involved. If she fills in the word or sound correctly, be sure to give her a rewarding response, like enthusiastically saying, "That's *right*, Winnie the *Pooh*. Good talking!" Repetitive songs like "Old MacDonald" are great too. When you get to the animal sound, pause and see if your child can fill in the blank.

Making It Funny

By the end of their first year, babies usually begin to develop a sense of humor and may be surprised or amused if you make up silly new verses to favorite songs. For example, when singing "The Wheels on the Bus" you could sing, "The cows on the bus say moo, moo, moo," and then stop and say, "Wait a second! Cows on a bus? That's silly!"

 ## 3. THE COLOR SIGHTING GAME

Using Crayons

For an older child who has learned some of his colors, you might try handing him a box with a few crayons in it and having him give the person next to him a crayon every time he sees something of that color, like a red car or a brown car or a white building. If you're driving the car and someone is sitting next to him in the back seat, he can hand them to that person; if you're sitting next to him on a bus or train, that's even easier; he just hands them to you. An empty box means a BINGO and a nice treat or a tickle. Then you can put the crayons back and start again.

Using Color Cards

You can do the same thing with a small bag of color cards. One easy way to make a set of these is to take some paper paint samples from a hardware store and cut out some nice distinct colors—red, blue, green, yellow, black, white, purple, orange, and so on. If you think playing this game with multiple colors is too complicated, just put about five red color chips in a bag or hand them to your child and have him give one to the adult next to him every time he sees and points to something red. When he's given them all away correctly, he gets a reinforcer (perhaps praise followed by a small red treat, like a red Froot Loop).

4. PRETEND CAR OR BUS TRIPS PRETEND PLAY

You can use car or bus trips as a way to help your child understand pretend play by pretending to go on a car or bus trip just before or after you actually go somewhere in the car or on a bus or train. For example, when you come home from a short errand to the market, you can put the child in a laundry basket with a round object for a steering wheel and say, while pushing the basket around the room, "Let's pretend to go in the car [or train or bus]. Vroom, vroom! Here we go! What a good driver you are."

You can even set up a low table or shelf with some empty boxes of some of your child's favorite foods and help her pretend to shop for a few things. For example, you could push her in a laundry basket, saying, "Let's drive to the store! Okay, here we are at the store. Let's go shopping." Then help her out of the basket and walk past the shelf, saying, "Here are the Cheerios. Let's put them in the bag," and put them in a supermarket bag of whatever type you use. Do that with a couple more items, then say, "Okay, done shopping. Let's go home." Put her back in the basket with the bag and "drive" home. Then you might put her in her high chair and give her a few pieces of the type of food you just "bought" at the market. Remember, you're teaching your child to understand and enjoy pretending, so make this activity as much fun as you can. If she's confused or fussy, move on to something else.

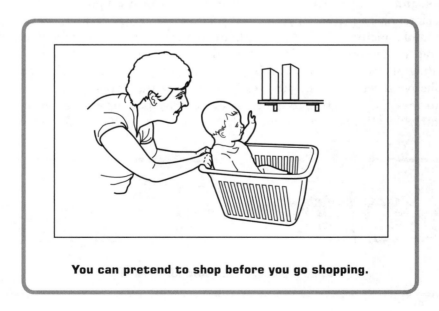

You can pretend to shop before you go shopping.

5. STOP AND GO   LANGUAGE

With the same activity, you can work on the words "stop" and "go." Use some construction paper to make a little red light/green light sign and help your child hold up the green paper or card as you say, "Green means go, go, go," as you push him or hold up the red card and say, "Red means stop," just before you stop the laundry basket car. If your child finds it fun, you can let him hold the two colors of paper; when he holds up green, you push him; when he holds up red, you stop. You can prompt him by helping him hold up the colored paper and then doing what it says, repeating "Green means go" and "Red means stop" each time. After you've practiced this for a while, you can begin to pause and let your child fill in the blank. For example, you can hold up the green "Go" sign and say, "Green means go! Ready, set, _____," and pause so that your child can fill in the blank and say "Go!," after which you can push him right away to reinforce him for saying "go." When you take your child on an errand in the car, you can use the same language on the car ride to point out real red and green traffic lights. When you get to a red light, point to the light and say, "Red means stop. The car stopped." And when the light turns green, point to it and say, "Green means go. Go, car, go!"

 6. PICTURE SCHEDULE FOR PLACES WE GO   THINKING/LANGUAGE

Another very good skill to work on when going on errands in the car is the idea of a picture schedule. The basic idea is to make a picture for each place you're going to go. Try to keep it simple, only two or three stops if possible. So if you're going to the bank and the supermarket, either make a picture or use a photograph of each of these places, plus a picture of your car if you're going by car or a bus if you're going by bus, and a picture of your home. Laminate them or just cover them with plastic wrap, taped down so the child can't get the plastic wrap off, or a sticky sheet of laminating plastic, which you can buy at a stationery or office supply store (called self-adhesive sheets). Put the pictures in a row (see the drawing below) and show them to the child, pointing to each one or holding them up for her to see, saying something like, "Look! First car [or bus], then bank, then supermarket, then home."

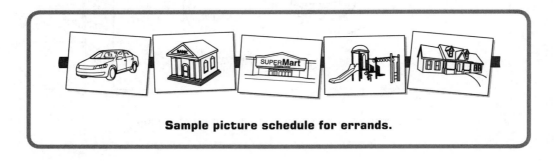

Sample picture schedule for errands.

If you can take your child to one of her favorite places, like the park or playground, after doing your errands, then place that picture after the pictures of the less exciting errands but before the picture of your house. So it might be pictures of car, bank, supermarket, park, home. Be sure to show the child the picture of each place as you get there, finishing with "Now we're going home. Yay! Now we're home."

The idea is to expose your child to simple language while reminding her of where you're going or where you went with the pictures and to help her develop the idea of doing a series of things. It may also help the child understand the order of her day, even though she does not yet understand all the language that she hears. If you have a picture of the fun place you're going to go after the supermarket, it might help her be able to wait more patiently in the market, but help her be patient by keeping each errand as short as you can.

7. THE ERRAND SONG   LANGUAGE/THINKING

As you leave for your errands, point to the picture, name the place you are going, and sing a song about it. You can do this after you review the whole series of places you're going. For example, if you're going to the bank, then the supermarket, then the park, you could show your child all those pictures and explain where you're going and then sing a song about the bank. For example, "We're going to the bank" could be sung to the tune of "The Farmer in the Dell." And if you use the same tune to sing a song about the market, the doctor, the park, or anyplace else, your child will soon become familiar with your errand song and may enjoy filling in the blanks with various place names when you point to the pictures of where you're headed next.

Working on "Hello" and "Good-Bye"

You can also reinforce your work on hello and good-bye. Each time you arrive and leave one of your errand locations, make sure to say "hello" and "good-bye"; for example, "Hello, bank!" and "Good-bye, bank!" If you can involve your child in any activity while at the market or bank, the errand will be less boring. For example, if you control your child's finger, perhaps you can let him push a button on the ATM or place favorite foods into the shopping cart at the supermarket. (If you hand him foods to put in, you can label the foods—for example, "apple," the word "in," or both: "Apple goes in, oranges go in," etc.) You can also play bingo by making your child a simple few squares of pictures (for example, cereal, apple, banana, juice), and each time your child spots one encourage him to point to and label it and then cover it with a sticker or check it off using simple language ("You found the apple! Only three more to go!"). Try to make it so that the last item your child finds is near the end of the shopping trip so you can give him a little treat (for example, an apple or a juice box) for "winning" the game. These types of activities will also give you extra opportunities to praise your child for being helpful.

8. REMEMBERING PICTURES OF PLACES LANGUAGE/THINKING

You can also work on remembering things by going over the pictures of where you went as soon as you get home. A very young child will not be able to remember where she was several hours earlier, but you can try this just after you arrive home, maybe while she is seated at the table or high chair having her lunch or a little snack. Put the pictures in the order you visited the places. For example, you might say while pointing to the pictures in turn, "We went to the market, and we got apples and cookies. Then we went to the playground. You went down the slide. Then we went in the car and came home." You can also keep a photo album and do this review on a weekly basis ("You went to Grandma's house and got a lollipop; you went sledding and it was cold!" etc.).

 ## 9. WAITING PATIENTLY BEHAVIOR/THINKING

A good concept to work on in the supermarket is waiting. Very young children won't be able to wait long without becoming restless, so don't ask your child to wait for more than a couple of minutes. You could pick up a favorite treat, like a package of chips or cookies, just before checkout, and say, "We have to wait a few minutes. After we pay, you can have a cookie." Then, as soon as you get through the checkout, open the package and give him a cookie for "nice waiting." If your child has trouble waiting for a few minutes and fusses to get the cookie, try teaching this by going to the market to get just two or three things. Think of this as a teaching visit rather than a shopping visit. Pick up the cookies and then head right for the express checkout, saying, "We have to wait; after we pay, you can have one." Make the waiting time as short as you need to get success, then you can lengthen it a little bit each time you visit the market.

 ## 10. STAY WITH ME BEHAVIOR

If your child enjoys being out of the cart at the market but tends to run off if you aren't holding on to her, here is a simple behavioral strategy that you can use to teach her to stay with you. Take along a small zipper bag with a special treat that your child enjoys, such as goldfish crackers or pretzels. Give your child the instruction "Stay with me" and prompt her to stay with you by holding one of her hands or having her hold on to the cart and closing one of your hands gently over hers. After a few steps, but before your child tries to pull away, stop briefly, praise her enthusiastically for staying with you, and give her a piece of her treat. Then give her the instruction to stay with you again and begin walking while she is still eating her treat. Add a few extra steps this time before pausing again to praise the child for staying with you and giving her another piece of her treat. Continue to do this, giving her the instruction "Stay with me" and adding a few more steps each time, before giving her a piece of her treat. Before long, you may be able to walk the length of an aisle, stopping to select items from the shelves and offering only one piece of the treat at the end of each aisle, without even having to hold on to your child's hand.

The more engaged you can get the child in the process of helping you pick up the items from the shelves and put them into the cart, the less likely that she will try to wander off. Even if she doesn't yet understand the names of the things you would like to buy, you can point to an item and prompt her to pick it up and place it in the cart. Then praise her enthusiastically for being such a good helper! Once she gets the idea and begins to enjoy this activity, trips to the market should get much easier.

11. FROM MARKET MATCHING TO VISUAL SHOPPING LISTS

THINKING/LANGUAGE/BEHAVIOR

Another way to use pictures is to work on simple matching. Let's say you're going to the supermarket and intend to buy a box of Cheerios and a carton of milk. Cut out the front of an old Cheerios box and the most colorful part of the front of an old milk carton. Then go down the supermarket aisle, letting your child hold the front panel of the cereal box or milk carton and look for the matching product. In this case, if he needs a prompt, the prompt would be to put him close to the product. As always, be sure to reinforce with praise when he finds the correct product. As your child gets better and better at matching you can use smaller pictures of the foods you're going to buy. You can find them on the Internet and print them, or cut the pictures used in newspaper ads or the weekly market circular. Below you'll see a little visual shopping list for six common foods you might shop for. You can hand them to the child one by one, when you're in the correct aisle, and make a game out of his finding the correct match and either pointing to it or lifting it up if it isn't too heavy and putting it in the cart or handing it to you.

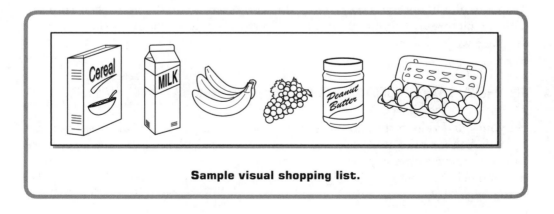

Sample visual shopping list.

For older children, you can even make a slightly longer visual shopping list, like six or seven items instead of two or three. By keeping children involved and engaged productively in the process of shopping, you will greatly reduce the likelihood of the problem behavior that is so common with children at the market. You can let your child know that if he stays with you and finds all of the items on his list he can have a treat. This works well for siblings, too. On page 105 is an example of a simple shopping list.

For a very young child, you want to make this easy by giving him one picture at a time to find, or you can point to the picture he has to find next and make sure you are near the item so it's easy to find. When the short shopping list is done, be sure to praise the child and, if possible, give him a small treat, like one chip out of the bag. This treat could be anything your child might enjoy, like something he tends to ask you for or want at the market. If he can wait for a few minutes, he can hold the picture of the chips until you get outside and then get a few chips as a reward. If the child is more mature and can wait until you get home, he can hold the chips until you get home (if it's a short ride) and then get a nice snack with his chips. But if he's too young to wait, just open the bag and give him a chip after he's gone through his very short list.

12. WHERE DOES BABY GO?   LANGUAGE

You can put copies of your errand pictures from your picture schedule into a small photo album for your child labeled "Where does Baby go?" (Use the child's name instead of "baby.") You could make a repetitive book out of it, like the ones we talked about before, and add it to your bedtime and naptime story collection. Using the same sentence starters each time you or your child turns a page will help her learn the place names. For example, the book may say, "Where does Baby go? Baby goes to the *park*." Or "Where does Baby go? Baby goes to the *market*." When you read the book to your child, put the emphasis on the name of the place. If you do this often, after a while you could begin to leave off the last word or pause and look at your child expectantly and see if she tries to fill in the blank. Later on, if you take the photo album with you on errands, you can teach her to "match" the real place with the picture by helping her flip through the book until she finds the picture of the place where you are.

13. HOW MANY ORANGES?   LANGUAGE/THINKING/EYE CONTACT

Let your child ride in the shopping cart. When you get to the produce section, get a plastic bag (or take along your own paper or reusable bag). Say, "Let's get three apples [or however many you want]." Hand the child one item (an apple, an orange, etc.) and help him put it in the bag while saying, "One," then count as he puts apples in the bag. "Two . . . three!!! You did it! You put three apples in the bag." Or, if you think he's ready, you count but pause for the last number, giving him a prompt if necessary: "One, two, three, f . . ." Or if he knows his numbers, help him recite the numbers, with prompts as necessary (a prompt could be placing your lips in the position to say "one" or "two" or "three" or giving him the first sound of the word). Then, to help him work on eye contact, hand him the piece of fruit, but wait for him to make eye contact with you before you let go so he can put it in the bag. If you need to, hold the piece of fruit up to your face to prompt eye contact. This game helps teach counting, coordinating his movements with yours, eye contact, and has the added advantage of keeping him busy. It will slow down your shopping a bit, but it's worth it if you can keep him engaged with you.

CHAPTER 11

Indoor Play

Indoor playtime is a wonderful opportunity to work on all kinds of skills, because you can be focused totally on the toddler, without trying to accomplish other tasks. Virtually any game or activity can be a great time to encourage eye contact by holding the desired object close to your face and reinforcing eye contact by giving the object to the child and by prompting him to communicate what he wants by pointing or speaking. Just remember to give the child as much help as he needs to be successful (even if that means hand-over-hand helping him point to what he wants) without upsetting him, because playtime should be happy time!

 ## 1. COLOR MATCHING AND COLOR WORDS   LANGUAGE/THINKING

There's at least one commercial game that has a large mat with rows of colored circles, but you can make your own by putting circles (or squares) of colored construction paper on the floor. Collect some brightly colored objects (red, green, blue, yellow, white, black) from around the house and put them on a table near the paper circles. Then hold up a toy and ask your child to put it on the colored circle that matches. Start easy by using two circles, with bright colors, so your child has to pick the correct one from just two choices. Then you can move to three or four choices. Teach your child to put the red object on the red circle, the blue object on the blue circle, and so on. You can use any objects that are brightly colored and easy to handle. As usual, give the child only as much help as she needs and fade your help as she gets the idea, starting with handing the object to her but keeping your hand over hers as you help her drop or place it on the circle.

You can also work on this in reverse (do whichever seems easier to you)—instead of placing the object on the colored circle on the floor, ask the child to pick up the correct circle and put it next to the toy or object. If she needs help, prompt her by walking her over to the matching circle and helping her pick it up and put it near the toy.

When she puts the object on the matching circle, or vice versa, give her enthusiastic praise ("You matched it!" or "You put the red ball on the red circle!") and give her a hug or a tickle or pick her up and swing her around—whatever she likes.

You can try to use objects that will also work as vocabulary builders. For example, if you're working on teaching your child the words for clothing, use small articles of clothing, like your child's socks, shirts, shorts, shoes, mittens, or hats. Or, you can even use doll clothing if you have it. Be careful to use only solid, primary-color pieces of clothing that are close to the color of the circles on the floor. You can do the same thing with toy cars, blocks, plastic cups and spoons, bath toy animals, like brightly colored fish or ducks, toy food items, or even some real ones. But really, anything will do. Just hand your child a colored object and say, for example, "Put the red apple on a red circle." If your child needs help, point to one of the red circles or walk him over to one of the red circles if she needs more help. When you praise your child, be sure to use the color word. For example, you might say something like, "Good for you! You found red!" or "Yay! Red car on red circle!" Another variation of this game is to begin mixing in verbs—for example, if your child has learned to identify some of the colors by name you could ask, "Can you hop to the red circle? Can you spin to the green circle?" Or use body parts: "Can you put your hand on the red circle? Can you put your foot on the green circle?"

As your child's language improves, offer her choices. For example, you might ask, "Would you like the green car or the green block?" To work on colors, you could hold up two blocks and ask, "Do you want the green one [hold it up higher or move it toward the child] or the red one [hold it up higher or move it toward the child]?" You can also just hold up the two objects and ask, "Which one do you want?" The child can make a choice by pointing or with words. If she doesn't make a choice, move the two objects close to her so she can just reach out and touch the one she wants. Label her choice with enthusiasm, for example, "You picked the green one!" Getting the object she chose should be a nice, natural reinforcer for having made a choice.

Once your child becomes good at matching and sorting primary colors, try experimenting with things that are different shades of the same color, like light green and dark green.

 ## 2. PUZZLE PIECE SCAVENGER HUNT LANGUAGE/THINKING/ NONVERBAL COMMUNICATION

Line up a small box, cup, and bowl. Make sure they are all empty and turn them upside down as shown on page 110.

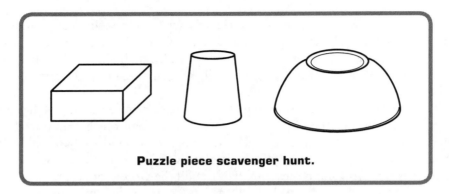

Puzzle piece scavenger hunt.

Choose a puzzle that your child especially enjoys and can put together easily. If he likes animals, you might want to choose an animal puzzle. Or, if he likes vehicles, a vehicle puzzle might be a good choice. Most children like the form-board puzzles when they are very young—the kind of puzzles with cut-out places for each piece rather than interlocking pieces.

Remove the pieces and hide one of the pieces under the box, one under the cup, and the other under the bowl and remember where you have placed each piece. If there are any remaining pieces, simply leave them in the puzzle board. Point to one of the empty spaces on the puzzle board—for example, the bunny—and say something like, "Uh-oh! The *bunny* is *missing*! Let's look *under* the *cup*!" Point to the cup if you think your child needs a little help or help him lift the cup if you think he needs more help. Cheer him on as he finds each piece in turn by following your instructions. Finding the pieces to one of his favorite puzzles will also be a natural reinforcer. This will help him learn the words for the animals or vehicles (bunny, car) or whatever the pieces show. It will also help him learn the meaning of "under."

You can do the same thing using the pieces of a Mr. Potato Head toy to work on body part vocabulary. You can say, "Oh! Mr. Potato Head needs his nose. It's under the cup." If he needs help, point to the cup or help him lift the cup. Then cheer him for finding the nose and help him put the nose on the potato head.

As your child gains more language, you can help him practice following simple directions by "hiding" things you know he will want. For example, you might place his blankie under the crib so that when he looks for it you can prompt him to ask, "Where's blankie?" and tell him, "I saw it under the crib."

 3. LOOK WHERE I'M LOOKING!   NONVERBAL COMMUNICATION/
SOCIAL ENGAGEMENT

In addition to working on understanding words ("It's under the cup") or understanding that you're pointing to where the piece is, you can use this game to work on helping your child *follow where you are looking*. Following your gaze and understanding what you're looking at is a very important skill for developing joint attention—that is, you and your child looking at the same thing at the same time—and it's also important for learning language. For example, looking at a flower while you say, "What a pretty flower" helps the child figure out what a "flower" is. You can say, "We need the car! I know where it is" or "We need Mr. Potato Head's nose! I know where it is." Then give an exaggerated look in the direction of the object where the car or nose is hidden. Spread the objects (cup, box, bowl, or whatever you're using) apart on the floor or a table so it's easier to tell which one you're looking at. At first you might need to point your whole head in the direction of the object. Make it really, really obvious. Then you can gradually make it harder by moving your head a little bit but moving your eyes to look right at the correct object. Of course, reinforce the child's finding the object you're looking at with enthusiastic praise and giving her the piece to put in the puzzle. If she doesn't look for the item where you're looking, provide a prompt by pointing to it, and if she still doesn't pick up the right object, help her pick it up and then reinforce enthusiastically ("You found it! Great! Let's put it in!"). These games—"Scavenger Hunt" and "Look Where I'm Looking!" can also be done with plastic Easter eggs, which are colorful and fun to try to find (especially with a little toy or piece of treat inside). You can say, "I see an egg!" and point to it, at first making your point quite close to the egg and later seeing if you can point from farther and farther away. You can also work on additional concepts, such as colors, rooms, and position words, with Easter eggs by hiding little treats in the eggs and telling your child that the treat is in the "blue" one or hiding in the "kitchen" or "next to" the table.

 ## 4. IT'S STILL THERE!   LANGUAGE/THINKING

Toddlers still love seeing object permanence in action; that is, they still get excited to see an object that has disappeared suddenly reappear. This is because very young children do not yet understand the idea that even when we can no longer see something it still exists. Show them how you can send little toy cars and balls through empty paper towel tubes and let your child watch as they come out the other side. You can put two or three of them together for added suspense or use an empty wrapping paper roll. You can also stuff tissues or scarves inside and take turns pulling them out again. Pop-up toys operate on the same idea. If you have a Jack-in-the-Box or another kind of pop-up toy, encourage your child to say "Hello!" as it pops up and wave "Bye-bye" as he pushes it back down. Start asking, "Where is it? Where did it go?" And then when it reappears, say, "Oh there it is!"

 ## 5. BUILDING BLOCK TOWERS   LANGUAGE

Very young children tend to really enjoy knocking down tall block towers—the taller the better! Help your child stack blocks into a tower. Sometimes children find it much easier to pick things up than to let them go, so your child may need a little extra help placing the blocks on top of the tower without knocking the tower over too soon. Use repetitive language to build the suspense, saying, "Build it up, up, up . . . and knock it . . . down!" Or, you could just say, "Up, up, up" as you stack the blocks, and then "Down!" as you knock the tower down. You can use the filling-in procedure here by doing this a few times and then letting the child say "down" as you or she knocks them down. If you think she's ready to say "down" or some approximation of it, you can look expectantly at the child and wait for her to say "down" before you knock down the tower or gently hold her hand to keep her from knocking it down until she says "down."

Some children will be frightened by the loud noise of the block falling on a table or a bare floor. If that's the case, just build a small tower of three or four blocks until your child gets used to the noise, then make it taller. If the tower falls before you or she knocks it over, say, "Boom! It fell down!" and make that fun too.

If you think your child is ready, try to introduce variations on the theme. For example, instead of saying, "Up, up, up," you could say, "It's getting taller, and taller, and taller! Look! It's SO TALL!" Or, if the tower starts to teeter back and forth, act very excited or scared and say, "Uh-oh!!! It's going to fall!" And, when you manage a *really* tall tower, try out the word "crash!" when it comes time to knock it down. Let your child participate in whatever way she wants to—by putting blocks on the tower, by knocking it down, by saying "crash," by completing "Ready, set . . . ," when you are ready to knock it down, or just by watching and enjoying. If your child is just watching you, you can still use the opportunity to work on eye contact by getting down on the floor and putting the next block briefly near your eyes before you put it on the tower or by putting your hand near your eyes as you say, "Ready, set . . . ," and then as soon as she looks at you, saying "go" and knocking the tower down.

 ## 6. PLAYING WITH BALLOONS   LANGUAGE/MOTOR COORDINATION/ EYE CONTACT

Helium balloons are another great way to teach the words "up" and "down." Make sure you have an extra-long string or ribbon attached to the balloon before you let it fly to the ceiling. Say something like, "Up, up and away!" as it flies upward. Then let your child reel it in as you chant, "It's coming down, down, down!"

Don't Throw a Partially Deflated Balloon Away!

As helium balloons deflate over a few days, they are great for playing catch or kicking because they move so slowly. You can throw the balloon toward your child a few times and let him catch it or pick it up. If he can throw it back toward you, great. If not, just get it from him and throw it again. After a few times, you can use this game to get eye contact. Stand near the child or even kneel down near him so it's easy for him to see you. When he looks at your eyes, praise him ("Great looking!") and immediately throw the balloon back to him. The balloon is the reward, and you are reinforcing eye contact.

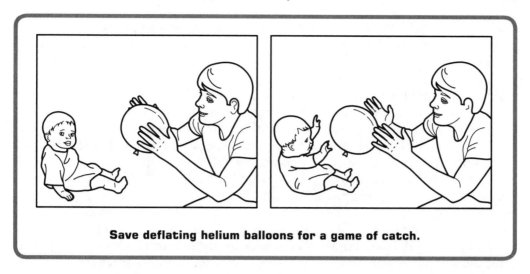

Save deflating helium balloons for a game of catch.

Using Regular Balloons

With regular balloons, try blowing them up and then letting them fly around the room by releasing them without tying them off. You can teach "One, two, three!" with the balloon by saying, "One, two . . . ," and then pausing before you say "three" as you let the balloon go. Or you could work on "ready, set, go." After you do this a few times, you can wait for the child to say "three" (or "go") and then reward him by letting the balloon fly. You can use this game to work on eye contact, too. The balloon flying around the room can make the child very excited, and some children find it easier to make eye contact if they are happy and excited and want you to repeat something. You can say "One, two . . . ," and then pause and wait for him to say "three" with even very brief eye contact and then let the balloon fly. If he has no words yet, you can say, "One, two, three," and then wait for eye contact before you let it go.

If your child picks up the deflated balloon, this might be a good time to help him hand it to you to play again or just hold your hand out as a prompt to get him to give it to you. **But note: *Never* let your child put the deflated balloon in his mouth—it's a choking hazard.** If he runs to pick it up after it flies around the room, be sure you are right there with him to keep him from putting it in his mouth. Of course, sometimes children are afraid of the balloon flying around the room because it makes a lot of noise and moves quickly and unpredictably. If that's the case with your child, you could try letting him stand across the room and blow up the balloon only about a third of the way before letting it go. If he's still afraid, just move on to something else.

7. LET'S PLAY BALL!   NONVERBAL COMMUNICATION, EYE CONTACT, MOTOR COORDINATION, SOCIAL ENGAGEMENT

Rolling a ball back and forth is a great introduction to turn taking, which is an important part of nonverbal communication and social engagement. It's easiest if you're sitting on the floor facing each other. Begin very close to your child so the ball doesn't have very far to go. Make sure you have eye contact with your child before you send the ball her way and then cheer her on for even attempting to get hold of the ball. **It will help a great deal if you can get a second adult to sit behind your child and prompt her to catch the ball and push it back to you.** There are some nice balls that light up or make music when moving, which might make the experience of rolling the ball back and forth especially fun for your child.

If your child is not particularly interested in passing a ball back and forth, you could try using a toy car or truck and put a small treat inside each time you push it to your child. Be sure to make a big deal of her as she finds the treat and takes it out of the car or truck, saying things like, "There's something hiding in there" in a sing-song voice and then, when she finds it, saying, "Yay! You found it!" or "Good for you! You found the yummy treat!" Be sure to keep the treat small (like one Froot Loop or even a half of one) so your child is motivated to keep playing. Then have the other adult help her roll it back to you so you can send another small treat her way.

Balls are also great for throwing into containers. You can begin with very large targets, like a laundry basket or an empty cardboard box, and gradually work your way down to something smaller, like an empty wastebasket or a children's basketball hoop. There are many that you can buy, very inexpensively, that will attach with suction cups to the wall or refrigerator. You might want to use a soft, lightweight ball that won't do any damage, regardless of how hard it's thrown. And your child might really enjoy your enthusiasm as you cheer her on when she makes the shot. Try doing a play-by-play to keep her engaged with you while she's throwing the balls into the various baskets. You can say things like, "She shoots! She scores!" or "What a shot!" "What an arm!"

 ## 8. FIND THE MUSIC   THINKING

If you have a music box, or any toy that plays music, hide it out of sight and then teach your child to follow the sound to find it. Start with easy hiding spots; for example, you could place it under a blanket right in front of him. Once he can find the source of the music right away, try hiding it farther and farther away so that it's a little more challenging to find it. Ask your child, "Where is the music?" Or say, "Let's find the music!" and then help him navigate toward the sound. Cheer for him when he finds it and dance or sing to the music with him. Once your child can do this without your help, try hiding yourself and call, "Where's Mommy?" from your hiding spot until he finds you. As soon as you make eye contact with him, say, "Here I am! Here's Mommy!" and scoop him up for a big hug and kiss.

 ## 9. MAKING MUSIC   NONVERBAL COMMUNICATION, LANGUAGE

Musical instruments, especially percussion instruments, are great for teaching the concepts of "fast" and "slow." And you can use almost anything, from a fancy children's xylophone to a homemade drum, which can be as simple as a small cardboard or wooden box. You can even have your child help you make a homemade shaker instrument by putting a handful of pebbles or dried beans into an empty water or juice bottle. **Note: Be sure to put some very sticky tape around the cap to prevent your child from unscrewing the cap and putting any of the pebbles or beans in her mouth.**

Put on some music or sing a song and play along. Give your child her own instrument that is similar to or the same as yours. See if your child will imitate you with her instrument and keep the beat of the music. If so, give her a big smile and continue singing and rocking to the beat. Try out different rhythms and praise your child enthusiastically for keeping pace with you. If she keeps a different beat, try to imitate her; if she is keeping a fast beat, you do the same; if she slows down, you slow down too. Either way, label her speed as either "fast" or "slow" and keep changing the label as she changes her speed. You can do the same thing with "loud" and "soft." Demonstrate loud banging, followed by soft banging, and label the sound you're making as either loud or soft. Try experimenting with different store-bought or home-made percussion instruments.

10. DANCE TO THE MUSIC   EYE CONTACT, LANGUAGE, SOCIAL ENGAGEMENT

Dancing around with musical instruments or ribbons or streamers can really bump up the fun. You can give your child some ribbons or streamers to hold, or you can attach them to a drumstick or a wooden dowel, and he can hold that. Put on some of your child's favorite music and dance around with him, waving thick ribbons or streamers as you dance. Dance in a silly, goofy way and then suddenly turn the music off and freeze with your finger on the play button. Wait for eye contact, and as soon as you get it turn the music back on. In relatively short order, eye contact will effectively serve as the on and off button for the music. You can also hold your child and dance with him, teaching him about the words "stop" and "go" by saying "Stop!" and then stopping the music every so often and freezing your dance and then saying "Go!" and then turning the music back on and starting to dance. Of course, if your child says "go" or "g" or even makes a sound with his voice while you are "frozen," be very excited, say, "Yes, let's *go*," and immediately start the music and dancing.

11. THE SINGING PUPPET   SOCIAL ENGAGEMENT

Sometimes even children who are not especially into music can have their hearts captured by silly singing puppets. So, if you're having trouble holding your child's attention with music, try having a puppet sing the song in a silly voice and see what happens. And if you don't have any puppets, you can make them. You can even have your child help you draw faces on an old sock or sack, a paper bag, or even your hand or thumb (see the drawing on page 116). Once you've made your puppet, have it sing to your child. Use the puppet to draw your child's attention to your face by

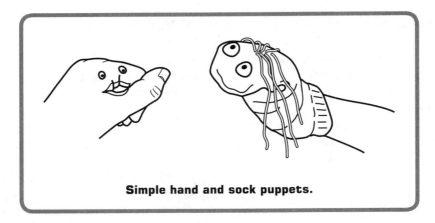

Simple hand and sock puppets.

having a silly conversation with the puppet. Hopefully, this will help her pay enough attention to you and the music that she'll realize how enjoyable it is to be a part of the fun.

 ## 12. FEED THE PUPPET   IMITATION/PRETEND PLAY

Once you have the puppet, you can work on simple imitation and pretend play by pretending to feed the puppet, or have it tickle the child's belly, or give the child a kiss, or ride in a toy car. Keep the action simple but make it dramatic enough to get the child's attention. For example, you could say, "Puppet [or whatever name you gave it] loves you. He's giving you a kiss." Then swoop in and have the puppet's mouth peck the child's cheek or the top of his head. Then have it tickle the child's belly or ride in the toy car. Then hand the puppet to the child and ask him to make the puppet ride in the car (or whatever you just did). If he doesn't do it, just gently help him with hand-over-hand help and say, "Yay! You made him ride in the car!" If he does, of course, give him even more enthusiastic praise.

 ## 13. ANIMAL TIME   LANGUAGE/PRETEND PLAY

It's great to have a "theme" for the day, as we described in Chapter 3. If you're working on teaching your child about animals, you could have a bag of toy animals and pull them out one at a time to play with. Hold one up to your face, such as a horse, and say, "Horse. A horse says 'neigh.' Horsie's going to give you a kiss." Then have the horse gallop up to your child's face saying "neigh" and give her a kiss. Then you could say, "Now Mommy's going to pretend to be a horse." Then go across the room and gallop over to the child, saying "neigh," ending with a kiss or a tickle. See if your child will join in, by pretending that she is the baby animal and you are the mommy animal. You can let your child choose another animal and repeat this with the animal she has chosen. Then line up different animals and sing

"Old MacDonald" and hold up each animal as you sing about it. After that, you can read a book about animals (like *Big Red Barn* or *Does a Kangaroo Have a Mother Too?*), watch a children's video or TV program about animals, play a matching game involving matching pictures of animal babies to their mommies (or if your child is not yet matching, try pretending the baby animal is going up to each grown-up animal saying, "Are you my mommy? No. Are you my mommy? No. Are you my mommy? Yes!"), or even go to a zoo or a farm or a pet store. Children love repetition, and having a theme for the day helps them focus on the new words and ideas.

14. THE VERY BIG BALL   LANGUAGE/EYE CONTACT/SOCIAL ENGAGEMENT

If you have a big exercise ball, try holding your child on top and bouncing him while reciting the first two lines of the "Humpty Dumpty" nursery rhyme—"Humpty Dumpty sat on a wall. Humpty Dumpty had a great fall"—and then making him fall forward and catching him or having him land in a pile of couch cushions and pillows as he "has a great fall." You could do the same thing with the chant "Trot, trot to Boston": "Trot, trot to Boston, trot, trot to town. Watch out, Baby, so you don't fall down!" When you say the words "fall down," make your child fall forward, either catching him or having him land gently on a big pile of couch cushions and pillows. If your child enjoys bouncing on the big ball, keep the bouncing going as long as your child remains engaged and looking at you. But just as you do with a swing (see Chapter 12), if he stops paying attention to you, freeze the ball. When he looks at you again, resume your bouncing, singing, and chanting.

There are so many children's songs, rhymes, and chants that are simply more fun on a big ball. For example, you could rock your child forward and backward on the ball while you sing "Row, Row, Row Your Boat" or bounce him up and down while you sing, "The Wheels on the Bus," holding the ball still when it's time to make the hand movement.

15. I WANT THAT ONE!   NONVERBAL COMMUNICATION/EYE CONTACT

Just as you do with mealtime, you can encourage eye contact and pointing by using small toys that the child likes, placed in clear plastic containers that the child needs help opening or that are in sight but out of reach, such as up high on a shelf. For example, you could put a small spinning top in one Tupperware container and a small animal figure in another. Put them in front of the child. When your child reaches for the one she wants, help her make a point with her index finger and point to the one she wants, saying, "You want *that* one! Okay!" Then wait for brief eye contact, prompting that by putting the Tupperware next to your eyes. As soon as you get eye contact, open the container and give the child the toy. Let her play with it for a few minutes, then start again, taking the toy away and putting it quickly out of sight or putting it back in the Tupperware.

CHAPTER 12

Outdoor Play

The following are activities that you can do with your child at the park, at the playground, or in your backyard.

 ## 1. LET'S GO SLIDING!   LANGUAGE

Playing on the slide is a good activity for teaching the concepts of "up, up, up" and "down, down, down" as well as the phrases "Ready, set, go!" and the concepts of "together," "all by myself," and more. You can help your child slide in different positions, such as sitting up or lying down on his tummy or on his back, sitting on your lap, or going down all by himself. Each time you do one of these things, label it for him ("all by yourself," "Mommy and Baby together," "on your tummy," "sitting up," "on your back"). If he's old enough to go up the ladder by himself safely, you can even have him slide through the "Mommy tunnel" by standing at the bottom of the slide with one foot on either side. If you go up with him, at the top you can say, "Ready, set, GO" and on "GO," let go of him or even give him a little push (if he's big enough to go by himself) or slide down with him in front of you.

Try using repetitive language chants and the filling-in procedure to teach words like "up," "down," and "go." For example, if you go up the ladder behind the child, say, "We're going up, up, up" and on the way down say, "We're going dooowwwwwn." Use the filling-in procedure, saying "We're going up, up . . . ," and leaving off the last "up" for him to fill in. If he doesn't, just fill it in yourself. After you've labeled his sliding positions for several trips to the slide, begin offering him choices.

For example, you could ask, "Would you like to sit or lie down?" or "Do you want to go together or all by yourself?" If your child doesn't answer, simply prompt him to choose the one you think he might like best: "Okay, let's go together." When he's at the top, you can say, "Now you're UP . . . ," and then when he slides you can say, "You're DOWN!" Or when he's at the top you can say, "Far . . . ," (with a rising intonation) and then when he comes down say, "Near!"

For a child who is comfortable sliding on his own you can also play "peeka-boo" by hiding under the slide and then jumping out to surprise him. Another silly game is to sit at the bottom of the slide facing away from the child and pretend you have no idea where he has gone ("Where did my baby go?") and then when he slides down and you get a gentle bonk as his feet touch you, you can say, "Oh, there you are!" Of course, any time he tries to fill in with words, or indicates what he wants in another way such as looking at you or pointing, be sure to honor his request enthusiastically.

2. SLIDING WITH FRIENDS   SOCIAL ENGAGEMENT, BEHAVIOR

If you're at the park or playground with other children who are also playing on the slide, this can be a nice opportunity to work on waiting patiently and taking turns. If your child has difficulty waiting her turn, you can practice when you have the slide to yourselves, by having your child's stuffed animals take turns with her sliding down the slide. You can announce each stuffed animal's turn, as well as your child's turn, saying, "Teddy's turn, Elmo's turn, Baby's turn!" Be sure to make the stuffed animals climb up the ladder to the slide, but make their turns relatively quick so that your child doesn't have to wait very long for *her* turn. Praise her for "Nice waiting!" after each of her stuffed animals takes a turn, and just before her turn say, "Great waiting!! Now it's *Baby's turn*!" This way her turn to slide is a natural reinforcer for waiting nicely and taking turns. Over time you can make the stuffed animals take slightly longer turns so the child has some practice waiting about as long as she would for another child to have a turn. Then you can begin to let her practice taking turns with one other child at a time, praising her heartily for being such a good turn-taker.

3. LET'S GO SWINGING!   EYE CONTACT/NONVERBAL COMMUNICATION/LANGUAGE

Pushing your child on the swing is one of the best and easiest activities for improving your child's eye contact. Stand in front of your child and give him a few good pushes from the front, to get him going. If he is looking at you and sharing the experience with you, keep it going. When he looks away for more than a few seconds, gently catch the swing with both hands, hold it still, and wait until he looks at you before pushing again (see the drawing on page 120). Give him a big smile and say

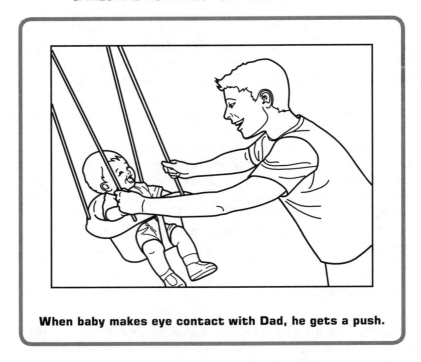

When baby makes eye contact with Dad, he gets a push.

"push" as you begin pushing. Repeat this for as long as your child is enjoying it. It might help if you sing a song with him about swinging while he is swinging and then suddenly stop singing when the swing stops swinging. One song you can use is "Swinging up and down in my great, big swing [three times], Won't you be my darling?" to the tune of "Skip to My Lou." Resume your singing and pushing when you get eye contact from your child.

Over time, your child should look at you for longer and longer periods, **sharing the experience with you** instead of just enjoying it by himself. And he should learn that looking at you is a way of communicating with you. Then you can also begin to work on expanding his communication by prompting him to add a word or sign, like "push" or "go," to the eye contact before you push him again. If your child can't yet speak, prompt a hand sign (see the drawing on page 121) or a gesture such as pushing outward in a pushing motion with one or both hands. Of course, you'll want to be sure he's holding on tight again, before you give him a push. This is true even if he is in a toddler safety seat, because eventually you want him to be safe on the swing when he is swinging all by himself.

Your child might find it funny if you pretend that he's knocking you down by letting his feet just touch you as he swings toward you and then falling back in an exaggerated way, saying, "Bonk!" Or you can duck out of the way as he comes toward you, saying, "Whew!" and pretending each time that you just barely escaped being knocked over.

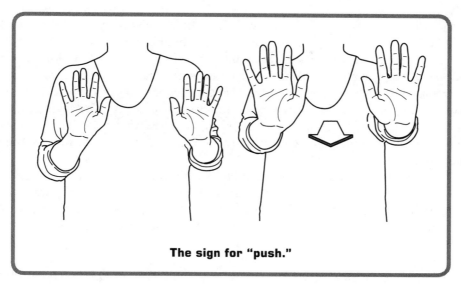

The sign for "push."

4. DRAWING WITH SIDEWALK CHALK   IMITATION/THINKING/MOTOR

First, just let your child make any mark she can and praise her for it. If you're working on shapes, draw several circles, point to one, and say, "Circle. What else could it be? It could be a sun." Then draw rays of sun around the first circle. See if your child can draw the rays of the sun around the next circle. If not, you can help her. Don't forget to praise her ("Great drawing! You made a sun!"), even if she needed hand-over-hand help.

Continue to draw other simple pictures, beginning with the other circles that you've drawn. For example, say, "This circle could be a balloon." Draw a tail and string on the second circle. Or, "It could be a face." Draw eyes, nose, and a mouth. Then point to each picture you have drawn and show your child how each one is round, saying, "A sun is a circle, and a balloon is a circle, and a smiley face is a circle," and so on.

5. BUBBLES, BUBBLES, BUBBLES!   EYE CONTACT/NONVERBAL COMMUNICATION/ IMITATION/MOTOR SKILLS

Bubbles are great fun but also excellent for working on eye contact and requesting. Blow a string of bubbles and encourage your child to chase after them or pop them. Do this repeatedly, making a really fun game of it. As soon as you can see that your child is really enjoying the game, hold the bubble wand to your lips, pause, and look expectantly or questioningly at your child. As soon as he looks at your eyes, say "Bubbles!" in a happy tone of voice and blow another string of bubbles for your child to enjoy. If you need to help him make eye contact, bring the bubbles and wand slowly up to just next to your eyes, to make it easier for your child to look at you as he looks at the bubbles. You can play the bubble game for a long time, with a lot of opportunities for getting eye contact, because most children don't get tired of bubbles very quickly. And once your child is good at making eye contact with you as you play with bubbles together, you can begin to work on teaching him to request the bubbles by pointing while he's making eye contact or by saying the word "bubbles" or even the "b" sound. Just prompt and reinforce whatever you want your child to do and then fade your prompts over time until your child is asking you to blow more bubbles all by himself.

If your child wants to blow the bubbles by himself, show him how. Show him how you form your lips in a tiny "O" shape before blowing. If he really wants to do it, this might encourage him to pay close attention to your mouth so that he can try to imitate you. Of course, make sure he doesn't put the wand in his mouth.

 ## 6. SAND AND WATER   LANGUAGE/THINKING/EYE CONTACT/
NONVERBAL COMMUNICATION

Take a bag of small plastic toys to a sandbox or sand table. Little plastic character toys or action heroes or even small toy cars or trucks will work well for this. Hide one or two toys in the sand. For example, take out a blue car and a red car and hide them in the sand. Then turn your palms upward and with a confused look on your face ask, "Where did the red car go?" Then help the child dig in the sand and say, "Oh there it is! We found it! We found the red car! Hooray!" When this game gets too easy for your child, you can make it more complex by placing a toy in a cup of damp sand and then making a little "sandcastle" with the toy inside. Then make some other cup sandcastles without a toy inside. Ask your child, "Where is the toy? Is it here?" Then help him "stomp!" on the first castle and see if the toy is there: "No; is it here?" (Help him "stomp" on the next one.) "Yes!"

You can use most of the same repetitive language routines that we talked about for the bath (see Chapter 8) either in the sandbox or at the water table. Sand and water are great for scooping and pouring, and there are some very nice water wheel toys that work well with very dry sand too.

If your child enjoys pouring water or sand in and watching how the wheels turn, you can easily work on eye contact by keeping control of the scoop or paper cup, filling it with sand or water, waiting for brief eye contact (putting the scoop near your eyes to prompt eye contact if necessary), and then handing it to your child so that *she* can pour it in. Just wait for eye contact before handing her the filled cup, scoop, or shovel.

You can use this toy to work on requesting and making choices as well as teaching colors, big and little, and many other things. Just use your imagination. For example, fill a big cup and a little cup with water and ask your child which one she wants to pour into the water wheel. Wait for her to point to the one she wants or to reach for it if she's not yet pointing. Or, if she says some words, prompt her to say "big" or "little" by demonstrating those words or just giving the child the first sound. If she says or tries to say the word, praise her for good talking and give her the one she requested.

You can do the same thing with red and green shovels that are filled with sand. Hold up both shovels and wait for your child to reach, point, or say "red" or "green," depending on what she can do. The possibilities are really endless. As long as your child enjoys playing with the toy, you can teach her all kinds of things using the toy as the reinforcer and waiting for her to make eye contact, point, reach, or speak, depending on what you want to work on and what she can do.

7. MIXING COLORS AT THE WATER TABLE OR THE SINK

THINKING/ NONVERBAL COMMUNICATION

You can also fill paper or plastic cups or bowls with water and different drops of food coloring. Let your child mix and pour them together and watch the colors blend together. You can offer him choices of the colors by holding up two different bottles of food coloring and asking him to show you which one he wants by saying the color or pointing or, if he's not yet pointing or speaking, by making brief eye contact with you and reaching for the one he wants.

8. MORE WATER PLAY

LANGUAGE/IMITATION

Water play is just plain fun, especially when it's warm outside. Use a sprinkler or wading pool to reinforce your "wet and dry" routines from bathtime (see Chapter 8). You can work on motor imitation and action words too. For example, you can say, "Follow me! Let's jump through the sprinkler. Now let's crawl through the sprinkler. Now let's run through the sprinkler," and so on. Add a little song if you think that might add to your child's enjoyment. For example, to the tune of "The Farmer in the Dell" you could sing, "We're crawling through the sprinkler. We're crawling through the sprinkler. Hi Ho the Derry-O. We're crawling through the sprinkler."

Use a hose and a big bucket of soapy water to wash your car or your child's toys, singing, "This is the way we wash the car, wash the car, wash the car. This is the way we wash the car. To make it clean and shiny."

9. WATERING CAN SPRINKLING

LANGUAGE

You can teach lots of language as you fill a watering can with water from a hose or at a sink and then walk around the yard watering all kinds of plants. Turn the water on and off a few times as you fill the watering can, saying, "Now the water is on. Now the water is off. On. Off. On. Off." Draw out the words "on" and "off" as you turn the water on and off. If your child likes to watch the water pour into the watering can, turn the water off and then pause and look expectantly at him before you turn it back on again. Reinforce any attempt at communication, such as eye contact, pointing, or saying "on," by turning the water back on again.

Fill and empty a small watering can or children's pail using the words "full" and "empty." Use a repetitive language approach, saying, "Now it's full! Now it's empty. Oh no! The water is all gone! It's empty. We have to get more water!"

You can teach the names of all kinds of things that grow in your yard or nearby, singing a repetitive language song to the tune of "The Farmer in the Dell." For example, when you're watering a tree, you can sing, "We're watering the tree. We're watering the tree. Hi Ho the Derry-O, we're watering the tree." Try using the filling-in procedure (pause and wait to see if your child tries to fill in the missing word) to see if your child is learning the words like "tree" or "flower" as you repeatedly use them.

 ## 10. SCOOTER, WAGON, TRICYCLE, TOY CAR   LANGUAGE/EYE CONTACT

Push or pull your child around in a vehicle, making car sounds like "vroom, vroom" and "beep, beep." You can play the same games described in Chapter 9 using a laundry basket as a vehicle. Try making little cards for green light and red light; when your child holds one up, say, "Green light—go, go, go," or "Red light—stop!" If your child doesn't hold one up by herself, you can prompt her by gently helping her hold up a card and then responding as if she had done it by herself.

If you pull instead of push, you can face the child while you pull her. Then you can pause for a moment and wait for eye contact to start pulling again. Make it easy for the child to look at you, if necessary, by putting your face right in front of her; when she looks at you, say, "Nice looking! Let's ride again!"

PART III

GAMES AND ACTIVITIES FOR BABIES AT RISK

CHAPTER 13

0–3 Months

Congratulations on the new baby! At this point, your baby doesn't have much control over his own behavior, but he is still learning important things about the world and other people.

WHAT NEWBORNS ARE LEARNING

That They Are Safe

The emotional bond that typically forms between infant and parent or other caregiver during the first year of life (see Chapter 2) not only stimulates brain growth but also affects personality development and acts as a model for future relationships. In other words, during the first year your infant will (unconsciously) learn from you that people are good and reliable and nurturing and that the world is a safe place in which he can expect his needs to be met. Neuroscientists now believe this basic attachment is such a primal need that there are networks of neurons in the brain dedicated to it.

In addition, during early infancy the hypothalamic–pituitary–adrenal (HPA) axis, a human endocrine system that regulates our ability to respond to stress, affects our moods and emotions, and even influences how well our immune systems work, is continuing to form and is highly influenced by our early experiences. If a baby develops in a highly stressful environment, her HPA axis will learn to produce large amounts of cortisol and to initiate a "fight-or-flight" response at the drop of a hat. (Research has shown that nonresponsive adults are highly stressful for infants.) Conversely, by providing a calm, stable, and safe environment, in which we regularly attend to and soothe our babies when they cry and respond to them in a predictable way, we can help their bodies learn to produce the healthiest amount of cortisol and can help set their baseline mood as a positive one. In essence, the best thing you can do to optimize your child's brain development during the first few months of life is to focus on developing a close relationship with her in which she feels safe and cared for and to ensure that when she is not in your care she is with warm and responsive adults.

That They Are Loved

Studies done on infants in large institutions, as well as those left in hospital incubators early in life, taught us that, regardless of caloric intake, babies will actually not grow (called *failure to thrive*) in the absence of loving touch. This underscores how critical human touch is for optimal infant development. Studies have also been done with premature infants, which have shown, for example, that if infants are undressed for a full-body gentle massage by their mothers four times a day for 1 month, and rocked and snuggled for 5 minutes at the end of each massage, they will experience more weight gain, fewer medical problems, greater attachment with parents, and greater cognitive and neurological development compared with infants not given this opportunity to be touched.

More and more tiny babies are spending much of their days alone in car seat carriers, bouncy seats, and strollers, without access to human touch, and this is something we want to minimize in the at-risk infant. One reason that touch is so important for newborns is that their bodies are still unable to regulate themselves independently. For example, a parent or other caregiver's heartbeat provides cues to the infant's body about how quickly to breathe and when to sleep, while the smell of the adult provides cues to the infant's body for when and how many hormones to produce. In other words, the physical presence of others is necessary to help regulate a baby's developing systems. In addition, a baby who is in touch with a parent or other caregiver is usually most likely to be calm, alert, and in the optimum state for observing and processing all that is going on around him.

Every hug, every playful squeeze, every kiss and caress gives the baby tactile stimulation. With his body pressed into yours, he learns proprioception—an awareness of his own body and his body's place in space. He gets auditory stimulation from your gentle explanations, whispers, and songs. When carried, the swaying and the rhythmic rocking of his body stimulates his vestibular system, giving him a sense of balance and a secure feeling in space. He receives olfactory stimulation with the scent of familiar adults, and if he nurses he receives gustatory stimulation with the changing taste of his mother's milk. He has a great view when carried upright and is treated to varied visual stimulation as he takes in the sights of the world. He even gets movement stimulation as you change position when carrying him.

Moreover, the newborn is beginning to integrate perceptions—in other words, to recognize that the voice he hears, the body he feels, and the face he sees all belong to one person. Infants need lots of simultaneous visual, tactile, and auditory input to put these ideas together. Perhaps most important, the baby assures himself that all is well largely through the messages he receives through his skin, his largest organ. Being held in your arms helps to maximize your newborn's opportunity for happiness and other positive emotions, and because the infant is developing his baseline levels of the neurotransmitters that regulate mood, experiencing these emotions as frequently as possible may have a lifelong impact on his mental health. All of these different opportunities for learning create the stimulation for the neurons in the baby's brain to grow and branch out and meet and intertwine with other neurons. The more these neurons grow and branch out, the greater the brain growth. In short, humans literally require a great deal of physical touch to develop to their optimal potential.

THE COLICKY BABY

All newborns cry a fair amount, but 15 to 25% of newborns cry a lot more than others. When these otherwise healthy babies cry excessively and inconsolably for no apparent reason—they're not sick, hungry, wet, tired, hot, or cold—pediatricians call that colic. Pediatricians generally use the "rule of threes" to determine colic: crying bouts that start when a baby is about 3 weeks old (usually late in the day, although they can occur anytime), lasting for more than 3 hours a day, on more than 3 days a week, for more than 3 weeks in a row. It typically peaks at 6 to 8 weeks and subsides by 3 to 4 months. Colic isn't a sign that your baby is sick (although things such as reflux, food allergies, and exposure to cigarette smoke can cause further aggravation and tears). Nor is it a sign that your baby has belly pain, although the way she grimaces, clenches her body, arches her back, pulls her legs up, and screams till she's purple can make it seem so. Colicky babies can be gassy. But pediatricians now believe that crying causes gas, rather than the other way around, because babies swallow air when they cry. One way to tell whether your baby is in pain or has colic is to observe the way various forms of distraction help or do not help. Pain will not go away when you turn on the hairdryer or go for a ride in the car, so if you can successfully find ways to distract your baby, you can reassure yourself that she is not in pain.

Why some babies experience colic and others don't remains a mystery. Some doctors view it as a natural developmental stage that babies can go through as they adjust to all the different sensations and experiences that come with life outside the womb. Others attribute it to an imbalance of bacteria in the gut. Yet another theory is that colic stems from an imbalance of the brain chemicals melatonin and serotonin. Colicky babies might have more serotonin, which makes intestinal muscles contract. (One reason colicky babies can fuss more at night, this theory hypothesizes, is that serotonin levels peak in the evening.) According to this theory, the chemical imbalance naturally resolves when babies start making melatonin on their own between 3 and 4 months.

Although it's not yet clear what the source of colic is, it is clear that colic is *not caused by parental behaviors of any kind*. Of course, colic can take a toll on new parents. Excessive infant crying is associated with postpartum depression.

Don't hesitate to enlist help and take breaks from your baby. It's very important to protect your own physical and mental health. **Colic is very difficult to deal with, and the most helpful reminders to give yourself are: (1) there is probably nothing wrong with your baby when he is crying, and (2) the excessive crying is almost certainly temporary.** Luckily, colic does not at all relate to the type of temperament or personality your baby is going to have.

In terms of calming techniques, Dr. Harvey Karp advocates experimenting with "The Five S's": **s**waddling (the close quarters of a car seat can also act as swaddling), "**s**shhhhh"ing loudly in baby's ear (other types of "white noise" such as hair dryer, radio static, or fans, may also help), **s**winging baby (some babies respond better to large arcs when swinging them, some babies respond better to wind-up swings, etc.), allowing baby to **s**uck on a pacifier (sucking is calming and organizing for infants), and laying her on her **s**ide or **s**tomach (across your forearm or lap with her head resting in your hand so as to keep pressure on her stomach). A lot of parents have also reported success with vibration—whether taking baby for a car ride, seating her on top of the dryer (well supported, of course), clipping a vibrating toy to her crib, or purchasing a baby seat that vibrates. Some parents report that keeping the baby close to their body, in a baby sling or front carrier, for example, is also helpful. These techniques may or may not work, and they work some of the time but not all of the time; what works is largely about trial and error.

If you have any doubt about whether your baby is really in pain or has something other than the usual colic, be sure to consult your pediatric health provider.

What to Pay Attention To

We know that typically developing infants are born with a tendency to pay attention to human faces and voices above any other sights and sounds. Moreover, infants prefer infant-directed speech (sometimes called *motherese*), which is simplified, sing-song, and somewhat high-pitched, over other types of speech. They also prefer speech in their native language (which they began to be exposed to in the womb), and the voices of their parents over the voices of strangers. Infants prefer live voices (of even the most terrible singer) to recorded voices (of even the most wonderful singers).

Newborns like to look at faces that make eye contact with them rather than other faces and learn to recognize their family members relatively quickly despite their limited visual abilities (newborns can see only 8–12 inches away from themselves). Moreover, even newborn infants begin trying to direct their eye gaze to where their parents are looking and begin trying to imitate their parents' facial expressions. However, we don't know how these preferences may be altered in infants with special needs. Therefore, we believe it's important to provide the infant who may have special needs some extra practice to ensure that he preferentially attends to faces and voices as soon as possible. Infants will come to appreciate and expect what they are exposed to, and they learn to do this by repetition.

In other words, while it is important that all babies experience a great deal of eye contact and speech directed at them, it is probably especially important in the case of infants with special needs or when there is concern about an infant's development, that the infant receive even greater amounts of social input. **Other people will be the greatest source of learning for your child throughout his life, and the sooner he learns this, the better.** Although repetition will teach infants what to expect and what to attend to, infants will also pay attention to anything that is unexpected or out of the ordinary. You can use this information to capture your child's attention by providing regular doses of novelty within the safety and predictability of daily routines.

THINGS TO WATCH FOR

Each child develops at her own pace, but talk to your baby's doctor if your 1-month-old:

- feeds slowly or doesn't suck well,
- doesn't seem to focus her eyes or watch things moving nearby,
- doesn't react to bright lights,
- seems especially stiff or floppy, or
- doesn't respond to loud sounds.

Talk to your doctor if your 3-month-old:

- can't support his head well,
- can't grasp objects in his fist,
- can't focus on moving objects,
- doesn't smile,
- doesn't react to loud sounds, or
- ignores new faces.

HOW YOU CAN HELP YOUR NEWBORN LEARN

With all that growth going on in the first few months of your baby's life, there are lots of ways you can help stimulate his social–emotional development. Of course, these are just a few examples and you don't need to try all of them. Use the ones that seem most interesting to your baby, and of course you should feel free to think up your own games and activities.

Here are some general principles:

- Respond predictably to your child and **keep him comfortable** to the greatest degree possible to facilitate a close relationship in which he feels safe.
- **Touch** him as often as possible in a way that he likes.
- Give him as many opportunities as possible to experience **rhythm,** from allowing him to begin to experience the daily rhythms of night and day, by allowing him to nap for longer stretches at night, and exposing him to sounds and daylight while he naps during the day, to dancing, singing, and rocking, to holding him close so he can feel your heartbeat, to affording him opportunities for sucking. Maximizing your child's early exposure to rhythm is one of the greatest early experiences you can provide.
- Engage in a lot of **face-to-face interaction** with your child involving **eye contact** and **social smiling.**
- Respond with big reactions when he shows emotion and repeat things that **draw out his positive emotions.**
- Integrate both **routine** and **novelty** into your child's day.

Following are some specific activities you can use during daily routines.

Waking Up/Bedtime Routines

 GOOD MORNING, TOES!

This is the time to start morning and bedtime routines. The very young baby will not yet understand your words but will appreciate hearing your voice and getting to know a routine with you. You can expand on these routines as he gets older. Say, "Good morning, toes!" and then kiss your baby's toes. Then say, "Good morning, feet! Good morning, hands! Good morning, tummy!" kissing each body part in turn. If he comes to anticipate what you're going to do, or smiles when you get to a specific body part, reinforce this by doing that body part again or with an extra tickle or smile or cuddle.

 GOOD NIGHT, TOES!

Dim the lights and move to a comfortable spot near where your baby will sleep. Softly say as you give kisses, "Good night, toes. Good night, knees. Good night, tummy. Good night, chubby cheeks. Good night, Baby." Choose three soothing songs that will be the baby's lullabies and always sing them right before nap and bedtime as you rock her. Then put her in her crib while she's drowsy but not asleep. If you prefer to rock her all the way to sleep before putting her down, that's fine, too.

Feeding

 KANGAROO CUDDLE

Provide skin-to-skin contact by partially undressing yourself and the baby during feedings regardless of whether you are nursing or using a bottle (although staying warm is always important, so be sure to wrap yourselves in a blanket if it's chilly). Holding an undressed baby against your bare chest (whether you are male or female) under a blanket is called a "kangaroo cuddle," and newborns cannot get enough of it!

 ROCK-A-BYE BABY

Use this opportunity to provide rhythmic input by rocking or singing to the baby. Think about children's classics like "Old MacDonald" and "Twinkle, Twinkle Little Star," as well as any adult songs you enjoy. You don't need to worry about your baby understanding the words at this point—and if you're not good at remembering words, just make them up!

 LOOK AT BABY!

Use this opportunity to provide the baby with a stretch of unbroken eye contact while smiling, cooing, and whispering to him. If you feel silly or can't think of what to say, try telling the baby the plots of your favorite movies, TV shows, and books— he will, of course, not understand what you're saying, but he'll appreciate the variation in the sounds you make and your tone of voice. Having time where he can simply look at your face is important for attachment and helping him learn social cues and the importance of attention to faces. When he looks back at you, reinforce this behavior with a big smile or a gentle tickle (in other words, with something he likes).

 CHANGE IT UP!

Use this opportunity to provide your baby with varied sensory experiences by changing small things during feeding time, such as the level of lighting in the room and the texture of the blankets you use. Make as many different funny sounds with your mouth as you can (clicking, tongue clucks, smooching, whistling, humming, blowing lips like a motorboat, etc.). Do whatever gets and holds her attention. If you're nursing, you can begin to provide the baby with variation in the form of the taste and smell of your milk by making sure you eat a varied and healthy diet. When you and other family members are eating, place the baby where she can see your faces, hear your voices, and smell the food.

WHAT DOES BABY NEED?

Practice trying to read the cues your baby gives you to let you know that he needs to be burped or moved into another position. Talk to your baby about the good times you've been having together and the good times ahead. (The more language babies hear during the first year, the more they will talk in their second year and beyond!)

Diaper Changing and Dressing

 FEELS SO GOOD!

Making sure to keep her warm, use changing time to give your baby some stimulation directly on her skin, such as a gentle baby *massage*. Using a milking motion, gently squeeze down each arm and leg. Then move your hands from her torso out to her sides, or draw shapes on her belly, then gently massage her temples in circles. You can do this with dry skin or with a bit of vegetable-based oil. Roll a small beach ball up and down her body, giving her a chance to experience a new type of tactile stimulation as well as practice grasping. Similarly, if you have a ball on a string, you can hold the ball over the baby while she reaches, kicks, etc. If she smiles or looks at you during these activities, reinforce this by saying, "Oh, you like that! Let's do it again," and repeating what she liked. And of course, if your baby expresses displeasure with any of this sensory stimulation, you should respond to what she has communicated and use even more gentle touch or stop altogether. The next time you try, remember to touch very gently and for only a very short time, increasing the sensory stimulation gradually over a period of days, weeks, or even months, as your baby comes to tolerate or even enjoy it.

 I CAN MAKE IT HAPPEN!

Sew little jingle bells on a pair of socks. Put the socks on the baby before changing time. You can let him explore the cause and effect of hearing bells when he kicks. Or crumple up tissue paper or cellophane and put it under the changing table cover, near his feet, so he hears crunching sounds when he kicks. On a special occasion, bring home a couple of helium balloons and let them go just above the baby's changing table so that the strings hang by his hands or you could tie them loosely around his wrists or ankles so that the balloons bump around when he moves his arms or kicks his feet.

 WHAT DO I SEE?

Change the baby next to a mirror so she can watch herself and begin to learn that she sees movement in the mirror when she moves (although she won't learn to recognize herself in a mirror until she's at least a year old). Or change her under a toy with something hanging from it that she can focus on, and, eventually, bat at with her hands, or underneath a mobile so she can watch it spin as she will be learning to track things visually. Hand her a rattle to shake while you change her.

 TUM-TUM ON THE TUMMY

Lightly "play his tummy" as if it were a little drum, keeping the beat while you sing to your baby. If he laughs or smiles or looks at you, give him a big smile, or a "yay" and a tickle or cuddle.

(Bathtime)

 JUST RIGHT!

Bathtime can be tricky for tiny babies if the air is too cold, the temperature of the water is not right, the pressure is too much while you wash, or they don't feel securely held and safe. Try to notice what aspects of the bath make your child either uncomfortable or happy and adjust for future baths. If she gets upset, the most important thing is to soothe her and make the bath more comfortable for her. If she looks at you and smiles, you can reinforce that with a big smile, a tickle or, if she seems to like the feeling of the water, you could gently pour some warm water on her tummy.

 LOOK AT ME!

Every time your baby makes eye contact with you, burst into a huge smile and praise him. Try to maintain eye contact as you wash him and tell him the steps of what you're doing. Think about whether there are any bath songs you can sing: "Rubber Duckie," or "Splish-Splash," or make up your own (e.g., to the tune of "London Bridge": "We are giving you a bath, you a bath, you a bath. We are giving you a bath, my fair baby"). When your baby looks away from you, pause your singing, and when he looks back at you, begin singing softly again. In this way, your baby's eye contact will be like the on and off switch for the music.

 WHAT DO I SEE?

Blow bubbles near the baby and watch for visual tracking. Make it easy for her to track the bubble by holding it close (8–10 inches away) and moving it slowly. Catch a bubble on your wand and hold it close so she can pop it by reaching or try popping it on her belly by moving it close. Hold up different bath toys near your face—once she focuses, slowly move either your head or the toy to give her a chance to practice visual tracking.

WHAT DO I FEEL?

Have lots of different textures handy for the baby to explore—for example, a sea sponge, a gauze sponge, a loofah glove, or a washcloth. You can also show your baby the properties of water by pouring water on him, drizzling water on him, and helping him splash. Kick baby's feet for him in the water, perhaps to a song (for example, to the tune of "Twinkle, Twinkle Little Star": "I am splashing with my toes. Look how far the water goes. I am kicking with my feet. Mommy thinks I'm awfully sweet," etc.). Poke holes in the bottom of a plastic bottle and fill it with water and then hold it up, letting the baby watch, and even feel, it "rain." If he laughs or looks at you, reinforce this by making it rain again while you cheer.

Doing Errands/Going for a Walk

 WE'RE GOING IN THE CAR!

When you go in the car, talk to your child in a sing-song voice about where you're going as you put her in the car seat. Wait and make sure you have her eye contact before smiling and begin singing a song where she can hear you. As you move away but continue to sing, she'll feel reassured that although you are in the front seat, out of sight, you're still nearby.

 WE'RE GOING FOR A WALK!

When you take a walk or run an errand, carry or "wear" your baby in a front carrier as much as possible. Try to direct his attention to exciting and colorful things along the way. Narrate what is happening using very simple language, pointing to things of interest and labeling them as you walk by. Frequently stop to gain baby's eye contact, and whenever he coos or makes a sound, imitate it to get his attention and reinforce his vocalization.

 LET'S WORK OUT!

Try to find safe ways to incorporate your baby into your exercise routine (making her fly like an airplane on your shins while you're lying on your back, giving her tummy time on your tummy while you do sit-ups, using her as a weight and lifting her slowly up and down with your arms). You can also add singing—for example, singing "Row, Row, Row Your Boat" while doing sit-ups or singing "The Grand Old Duke of York" (listen to it on YouTube) as you lift her up and down. If she smiles or makes eye contact while you're doing that, reinforce it by repeating the action she likes.

Chores around the House

 LET'S WASH THE CLOTHES!

When you do laundry, see if your baby likes being securely held in a baby seat on top of a vibrating washer or dryer. Of course, make sure the top of the dryer is not too hot. Talk to him and tell him each piece of laundry you're putting in the washer or dryer (of course, he won't understand, but hearing words for common objects in the first year will help his language development).

 I SMELL CINNAMON!

As you cook with baby safely in a carrier, periodically let her smell different items from your cabinets (cinnamon, basil, mint tea, etc.).

Playtime

 RHYMES AND SONGS FOR BABY

Say this rhyme as you trace baby's face: "Here's where the coachman sits" (make a gentle circle on his forehead), "here's where he pats his horse" (make another circle underneath), "eye winka" (trace one eyebrow), "eye blinka" (trace the other eyebrow), "nose droppa" (trace down his nose), "mouth eata" (trace his mouth), "chin chabba, chin chabba, chin chabba" (with a big smile, give a gentle tickle to his chin).

Chant these words as you gently move your child's legs "together, apart, together, apart, up, down, up down, zigzag, zigzag, to the left, to the right," then hide behind her feet: "Where's Mommy? Peekaboo!"

Touch your baby's head and say, "Here is north"; touch his feet and say, "Here is south"; stretch out both of his arms and touch or wiggle one, saying, "Here is east" and the other, saying, "Here is west." Then point to yourself: "Here is Mommy so, so happy" (ham it up with big smiles) "because here's the baby that I love best!" (swoop in for a hug or nose rubs or a kiss).

Try singing or saying rhymes with your lips pressed right up against his bare tummy.

Try singing the "name game" song with the names of everyone familiar to your baby. It goes like this, but of course make up your own silly name game if you prefer: "Jackie, Jackie, Bo backie, banana fanna foe fackie, me my moe mackie. Jackie!" Or "Mommy Mommy bo bommy banana fanna foe fommy, me my mo Mommy. Mommy!"

All of these rhymes and games are intended to get and hold your baby's attention. Reinforce his looking at you or smiling with a gentle "yay" and by repeating the rhymes and games that he liked best.

REALLY? YOU DON'T SAY!

When your baby begins to coo (usually around 8 weeks), find a comfortable way to rest face to face and try repeating the sounds she makes. You can also pretend she is telling you a very interesting story, saying things like, "Really? Oh my! Tell me more." Your verbal and facial responses to her sounds will let her know that she is on to something with this whole communication thing and that she should continue!

 A WALK AROUND THE HOUSE

Take the baby for a walk around your home and point out all the rooms and all the exciting (or ordinary) things in each room and what the rooms are used for, making a special point to stop at all of the mirrors and let him look at the two of you in the mirror. Reinforce eye contact in the mirror with a gentle tickle or hug (or whatever he likes).

 LET'S MOVE!

Put on some music and dance to the beat while you're holding your baby. Or sway the baby from side to side while holding her under her arms and chant: "Tick tock, tick tock, I'm a little cuckoo clock. Tick tock, tick tock, now I'm striking one o'clock [lift baby up to the sky once]. Cuckoo! Cuckoo!" Continue with two and three o'clock, lifting baby up two and three times respectively. Place your baby on a blanket and take him for a "boat ride" by slowly dragging the blanket around with him on it.

 LET'S LOOK!

Begin to help your child develop looking and visual tracking skills. Show her some black-and-white pictures—newborn babies love high-contrast images—and also lots of pictures of faces. Newborns also love (or should learn to love) looking at faces.

Try hanging a clothesline over the crib and rotating the objects you attach to it. You can move them on the clothesline and talk to the baby about each one, giving her visual and verbal input.

A variation is to hang things that make different sounds, such as a small bell, a rattle, or a squeaky toy. When you have her attention, perhaps while singing, begin to move or sway slowly to the left and then to the right. See how long and how far your baby can follow you with her eyes.

You can also blow bubbles and see if your baby will watch them float away.

Grab a puppet (or make your own with a sock; see the drawing in Chapter 11) or a stuffed animal. Make the puppet pop in and out of baby's sightline, for example over the side of the bassinet, from behind your back, or from under a table. If you create simple patterns, you can begin to watch your baby shift the direction of her gaze, anticipating where the puppet will next appear. (Another variation is to use a squeaky toy.)

Find some soft, brightly colored toys and move them slowly around the baby's visual field, sometimes giving her a light stroke with it on her tummy, arms, and feet, so that she can experience the sight and texture at the same time (a bag of brightly colored cotton pompoms or feathers works well). Pompoms can even be dropped onto your baby's tummy because they are so light. A variation on this game is to pretend your finger is a buzzing bee or your hand is a quacking duck and move them closer and closer to the baby until they land on her or touch her skin and then start over.

 LET'S TOUCH!

Give the baby practice grasping and banging by letting him explore objects such as measuring cups and spoons, as well as blocks and squeaky toys and cloth books. Cover each finger of an old glove with differently textured materials (making sure to secure each piece so that there are no choking hazards). You can use flannel, silk, velour, a large button, and so on. Your baby can explore the textures during cuddle time. Take a slotted spoon and tie some ribbons to it, then gently sway it back and forth above your baby so that he has something pretty to look at (before 2 months) and later something to bat at with his hands (2–3 months).

 LET'S LISTEN!

Place the baby on a blanket and touch her face and say "face." Then touch her hand to your face and say "face." Repeat this with eyes, nose, mouth, hair, belly button, toes, and so on, each time letting her feel yours after you touch hers. If she doesn't reach out (which she probably won't at this age), prompt her by gently guiding her hand to your body part.

 TUMMY TIME

Young babies need, but sometimes do not enjoy, tummy time, which helps strengthen back and neck muscles. Note: Sleeping, however, should always be on baby's back; tummy time should be supervised. You can see if your baby likes it when you place a rolled-up towel under his arms and chest to help him feel propped up. You can also try to make it more exciting in a few ways. First of all, you can also lie on your tummy facing the baby so that when he lifts up his head he sees you. Second, you can try to put interesting things right beneath him. For example, you might look for blankets with interesting textures (if you're feeling ambitious, you could even sew together a few different scraps to make a small blanket with a few different interesting textures or colorful patterns).

Another idea is to fill a giant zipper bag with water and a few scraps of colored paper or sequins, and then put the whole thing into another zipper bag so it's spill-proof. Show the baby that as the two of you push down on it, the paper or sequins will scatter in the water and the bag will change shape. If he makes an effort to push down himself, reinforce this exploratory behavior with a gentle cheer or cuddle and by helping him push down on the bag again.

Place him, on his tummy, on a small exercise or large playground ball while you hold him. You must make sure he feels very safe and secure that you are holding him and that he is not in danger, but as long as he feels secure, he will probably enjoy the sensation of being "rolled" forward and backward. As an alternative to a ball, you can roll up a towel or two to place underneath him while you roll him back and forth on his tummy.

Find a small plastic mirror you can put on the floor beneath him so he can watch himself. He will not yet understand that he is watching himself, but he will be intrigued!

Help your baby begin to track sounds by moving around the room as you sing and talk to him going near, and going far—see if he will turn his head toward you to keep his focus on you. For extra practice strengthening neck muscles, put the baby down on his tummy on a blanket in the middle of the room and slowly move in a wide arc around him as you sing to help encourage him to hold his head up and gently turn his head to follow you.

CHAPTER 14

3–6 Months

Three to 6 months is a period of rapid development. Your baby is starting to get more voluntary control over her movements, especially of the upper body, although she still has a very limited set of things she can do intentionally. She is feeling some different emotions now and starting to interact with other people in a deliberate way. Her biological rhythms are starting to be better developed, including when to eat and when to sleep.

WHAT 3- TO 6-MONTH-OLDS ARE LEARNING

At this age children are *continuing to learn* many of the things they started to learn in the first 3 months. The most important task for the 3- to 6-month-old infant continues to be to learn that he is safe and loved. He's still learning who his primary attachment figures or caregivers are, and his body is still taking cues from the environment to determine how much cortisol (stress hormone) to produce. (Is this a safe environment in which I can relax? Or do I need to be on guard all the time and scream to get my needs met?) Research is just beginning to investigate what happens when parents are trained in the kinds of techniques discussed here, and so far it has shown that providing infants with extra learning opportunities can improve parent–child relationships.

In most cases, colic (see Chapter 13), which can cause babies to cry and scream no matter what you do, will resolve by around 12 weeks (between 3 and 4 months) of age. If your child is still crying inconsolably after 4 months, it's important to talk to your pediatrician to find out whether your baby has an underlying medical condition (such as reflux, allergies, a hernia, or a urinary tract infection).

Babies of this age are also *beginning to learn* some new things.

141

Better Control over Their Bodies

Your baby now views the world in full color and can see farther away. She also begins to recognize people and objects from a distance. She is starting to recognize and distinguish different sounds. For a few months she will be able to make even finer-grained distinctions between language sounds than you can! After that, she will begin to lose the ability to distinguish between closely related sounds that do not have different meanings in her native language. This illustrates a principle that is important to think about when providing an enriched environment for a young child. Synapses or neural connections that are rarely activated during the first year—whether because of sounds never heard, textures never felt, or sights never seen—will wither and disappear. In some cases, most strikingly in the case of language, this process is important. By disregarding sounds that are unimportant to her native language, the baby will be able to focus her attention on sounds that are important to her language development. However, in other cases, such as sensory experiences, you want to help nourish and protect those synapses. You can do this by exposing your child to a wide variety of sensory experiences (for example, gentle massage, rocking and swaying to music, water play; in essence, as many different types of sights, sounds, tastes, textures, types of touch, and types of movement as possible), and in so doing assure that the brain remains maximally flexible and able to develop in a variety of ways.

By 6 months (although for some babies it's closer to 8 months) your baby will probably learn to roll on her tummy and back again, sit up without your help, and support her weight with her legs well enough to bounce when you hold her in a standing position. She will learn to pull objects closer to her and to hold them and move them from one hand to another. She will also begin to learn to coordinate her body movements—for example, shaking a toy and vocalizing at the same time.

How to Fall Asleep

It's time to begin establishing more of a schedule and routine for your baby. It's still too early to let the baby "cry it out"; however, you can begin to teach your child how to fall asleep by (1) not letting daytime naps extend beyond 2½ hours, (2) setting a predictable naptime and bedtime, (3) establishing a routine that signals your baby that rest time is coming (for example, sitting in a rocking chair, reading a story, turning down the lights, singing a lullaby and rocking the baby, or providing another type of soothing touch and then putting the child in the crib, bassinet, or bed very tired but still awake with some type of comforting object, like a favorite stuffed animal) and then remaining nearby until the baby has fallen asleep. Your baby's body will begin to use these cues to figure out when to produce the hormones associated with sleep.

Bedtime is the one time during which you do *not* want to make too much eye contact, because it is so stimulating. Similarly, avoid anything new or exciting or any screens (whether from a television, tablet, electronic reader, or mobile phone) or bright lights. Dial down the volume on sound and lower the intensity of visual and tactile sensory stimulation to create a soothing, relaxing atmosphere for your baby when it's time for sleep. No studies of infants and sleep have yet produced any meaningful differences between babies who sleep with their parents and babies who sleep in cribs, or between babies who are responded to during the night after 6 months of age and babies who are allowed to cry in the night after 6 months of age. The one clear difference that has been found related to sleep is that, by 1 year of age, infants who don't sleep well fall behind in their language and thinking relative to infants who do sleep well. Thus starting good sleep habits now is an important part of your plan to optimize your infant's development.

Beginnings of Social Interaction

Your baby is now beginning to fully engage with the world. He is smiling and will soon laugh and babble. He is now more sensitive to your tone of voice. Over the next few months he'll learn to heed your warning when you tell him "no" and begin to recognize his name and turn his head to look at you when you call him.

Although the infant needs to learn some things about the world that don't involve social interaction, social interaction is by far the most complex and the most important thing to learn about for future personal happiness. In addition, many of the other things he needs to learn can be taught within the context of social interactions. Your child is learning every hour that he's awake. Your goal is to have him learn about social interactions for as much of that time as possible. **That means setting up as many of the situations as you can in which your baby attends to you best throughout the day.**

During these months your baby will begin to learn how to play. The first types of play that typically engage children are sensory play and cause-and-effect play. Sensory play is any type of play that gives your child a unique physical sensation, either by changing his position in space, exposing his skin to different textures and sensations, or exposing him to different sights and sounds. Cause-and-effect play is any type of play that teaches your baby that when one thing happens something else follows it. For example, when you shake a rattle, it makes noise. The most important type of cause and effect for your 3- to 6-month-old baby to learn is that when *he* does something, something else will follow. This is the time when he begins to learn that he can have an effect on the world around him. When you respond *contingently* to your child (making your behavior and vocalizations dependent on his), you are teaching him about cause and effect and social interaction at the same time! For example, if you begin to sing a song or rhyme with finger plays every time your baby grabs your hands, he will learn that grabbing your hands is one way to get you to do this. If you smile at him every time he smiles at you, he will learn that smiling at you makes you smile. Even if his signals are not initially intentional, if you treat them as if they were intentional communication, they will become so over time. By making your responses contingent on his behavior, you're beginning to teach your baby that his actions have consequences for other people's behavior. Similarly, if you talk about the things that are the focus of his attention, or talk about how he's feeling and what he's doing, he'll learn language much faster. Research has shown that infants develop language faster and develop superior social skills when their parents interact and speak with them in a contingent manner.

Of course, you can't do this all the time, nor should you. Sometimes you'll be the one to initiate a social interaction by approaching your baby, picking him up, talking to him, or taking care of him (feeding, changing). But try to be aware of opportunities to respond to his behavior in a predictable way so that he can learn that when he does something (like touching your hands or smiling at you) you'll respond in a predictable and pleasurable way.

Asserting Their Individuality

All babies are different. It's important to pay attention to the situations in which your baby seems calmest, most alert, or happiest and the situations in which she seems overwhelmed, fearful, or frustrated, so that you can adjust the stimulation you provide based on your observations. For example, some babies become easily over-stimulated and will find it too much to have someone sing to them, rock them, and make eye contact at the same time. Babies who become overwhelmed by too much stimulation may love to be spoken to softly, to make forts or tents to play in, and may require a long time to get used to new things (for example, you may need to leave a toy out and visible for a few days before the child plays with it, or sing a song in the car several times before your child begins to enjoy it). Other babies may need a high level of stimulation to keep them engaged. For example, some children may seek out physical play, and actually pay better attention when there is novelty in their environment (for example, rotating your toys to keep them feeling new, having new people visit, or going to new places). Experiment with finding the right amount of stimulation to keep your baby calm and focused. At the same time, experiment with different strategies for remaining the focus of your child's attention. Do you find it best to place yourself strategically in your child's line of sight? To be the one holding the toys and objects of interest, sometimes near your face? Does your child consistently shift her focus to you when you begin to tickle or to sing? Start to take note of your "bag of tricks" for keeping your child's focus on you.

THINGS TO WATCH FOR

Each child develops at her own pace, but talk to your child's doctor if by 6 months your baby:

- seems very stiff or floppy,
- can't hold her head steady,
- can't sit on her own for at least a few seconds,
- doesn't respond to noises or smiles,
- doesn't smile when she sees a caregiver,

- isn't affectionate with those closest to her, or
- doesn't reach for objects.

HOW YOU CAN HELP
YOUR 3- TO 6-MONTH-OLD LEARN

Continue everything you did between birth and 3 months—respond sensitively and predictably to your child and give him lots of face-to-face time, eye contact, and language input. In addition, add the following pieces:

- Set up a variety of **sensory experiences** (textures, music, types of language, types of movement).
- Work on establishing a routine and schedule for eating, sleeping, and playing (routines are crucial to memory development).
- Use your child's name frequently.
- Set up a variety of cause-and-effect experiences. **Learn to respond to your infant contingently.**
- Learn about your child:
  - When does he pay attention?
  - When does he get overwhelmed?
  - What does he like?
  - What does he fear or dislike?
  - How can you make yourself the center of his happy attention?

We want to encourage babies to express a lot of positive emotion from as early on as possible. So find whatever games make your baby giggle (is it funny faces? certain animal sounds? being tickled gently?) and play them often.

Also keep in mind that babies of this age explore much of the world by mouthing things and make sure they have safe opportunities to do so.

Here are some specific suggestions for activities to do during daily routines:

Waking Up/Bedtime Routines

 WAKE-UP ROUTINES

One of the best teaching tools for infants is to create routines around daily activities like waking up and going to sleep. A routine is anything that has specific steps that are repeated often in the same order in which you and your baby each have a specific role to play. The routine itself is the important part, so feel free to create a different routine from the following suggestions.

MORNING STRETCH

"Stretch Mommy's arms!" (Do an exaggerated stretch.) "Stretch baby's arms!" (Gently stretch out baby's limbs.) Encourage baby to stretch her hands to her knees and her hands to her feet by helping to bring her feet up.

 MORNING GREETINGS

Say, "Good morning, [baby's name]! Good morning, ears! [Kiss ears.] Good morning, nose! [Kiss nose.] Good morning, belly! [Kiss belly.]" Open curtains and say "Good morning, sun!" Pick up your baby's stuffed animals one at a time and say, "Good morning, Elmo! Good morning, Pooh Bear!" Sing a "good morning" song like "Good Morning to You" or "Good Morning" from the show *Singin' in the Rain*. Reinforce any attempt that your baby makes to join in the game with a big smile and praise.

 READING TOGETHER

Try to read together every day. Begin with high-contrast books (with black-and-white or brightly colored pictures) as well as soft cloth books with different textures that your baby can explore with touch or books that your baby can play with in the bath or explore with her mouth. Try making it a part of your routine by reading before you sing a lullaby and put the baby down to sleep for naptime or bedtime. Hold the pictures up for your baby to see as you read. Point to objects in the book by touching your index finger to objects of interest. (You're beginning to teach your baby the meaning and significance of pointing. The first type of point he'll begin to understand is the point that involves you actually touching the object to which you want to direct his attention.) If you need to, draw his attention to your finger by wiggling it near him and then move it to touch the book while you say what you're pointing to. You can try to pause momentarily from time to time and wait for your baby to use his voice or body to get your attention (by making eye contact, vocalizing, or reaching)—this is the beginning of social turn taking! When he does this, reinforce this behavior with a gentle cheer or tickle and continue the turn taking by turning the page and pointing to and labeling something new and interesting.

 IT'S THE OPPOSITE!

Make use of your baby's desire to compare and contrast by trying to find a few "opposite" books that show almost the same picture but with one difference—for example, Elmo with his mouth open and Elmo with his mouth shut, a baby with a happy expression next to the baby with a sad expression, a dog soaking wet next to the same dog dry and fluffy, and so on.

NURSERY RHYMES AND LULLABIES

The rhythmic sound of nursery rhymes, along with the brightly colored books that usually accompany them, make another good early favorite for the very young child and can be repeated in the car and on walks. Sing a soothing lullaby before the baby falls asleep; choose a few different songs to be designated lullabies and don't sing them at any time other than before sleep. This way the songs will act as relaxation cues for your baby. Having a few different songs will mean that your baby will be familiar with each one but also get a bit of variety.

 SAY GOOD NIGHT

Say good night to the moon as you close the curtains, say good night to stuffed animals and give or blow them kisses, say good night to your baby's toes and fingers as you give them kisses, say good night to your baby. Continue to give your baby a familiar, comforting object, like a soft teddy bear or a small, soft baby blanket, or even an item of your clothing (sometimes called a transitional object), preferably one that smells like you if she is sleeping separately from you.

Feeding Time

 KANGAROO CUDDLE

Continue to make feeding time special by holding your baby skin-to-skin, in a quiet place, and making eye contact whenever possible. Reinforce eye contact with a soft cuddle or singing a song he likes.

 YOU DO, I DO!

A quiet feeding time is a good time to do quiet activities while you have your baby's attention. Your baby will begin to pay attention when you imitate her at this age. If she stretches her fingers wide, show her that you can do the same. If she makes a cooing sound, coo right back.

 HOW MANY TICKLES?

Your very young baby is actually able to distinguish small numbers (between 1 and 3), so, for example, you might try tickling him in sets of three—"tickle, tickle, tickle"—five or six times in a row. Then change it up and tickle him in sets of two— "tickle tickle"—five or six times in a row. You have begun to teach your baby about numbers! The same strategy of changing the quantity or rhythm can be applied to lots of different things such as swinging the baby three times before spinning, blowing three raspberries on his belly before smiling at him, or helping him kick his legs to splash the bath water three times. Reinforce his smiling and eye contact during these games by saying, "Nice looking! You like splashing! Let's do it again!"

LET'S TOUCH!

If your baby drinks from a bottle and is beginning to hold it, try placing different-textured socks over the bottom half as a "bottle cover" so that she has different textures to feel with her hands as she drinks.

Diaper Changing and Dressing

 BABY MASSAGE

Continue baby massage, but now you might begin to pair the music with your actions—for example, to the tune of "Here We Go 'Round the Mulberry Bush," sing, "This is the way we rub your arms, rub your arms, rub your arms." You might also begin to expand the number of textures and sensations you expose the baby to—for example, you can gently massage his bare skin, massage him with lotion, brush him with a soft brush, tickle him with a feather, tickle him with a silky scarf, or rub him with a soft blanket or washcloth. Try blowing on his belly, giving him raspberries, or whispering a secret to him (so he can experience the sensation of having whispering in his ear).

 GO–STOP!

Continue to let your baby crunch cellophane or kick with his jingle bell socks (see Chapter 13), but now begin to pair words ("jingle jingle") or music (singing "Jingle Bells") with her kicks, meaning that *you will speak or sing only when she kicks, and you will stop when she stops* (this is an example of responding contingently to her behavior), during this jingle bell play. Similarly, you can say "shake, shake" when the baby shakes a rattle or begin to sing a song. You may only sing for a few seconds before she stops kicking or shaking the rattle; then pause and wait for her to resume. If she likes this game, there are many ways to expand on it. You can wave your arms or dance around when your baby kicks or shakes and immediately freeze when she stops.

 WHAT'S COMING?

Begin to create *anticipation* with these games: Using a mirror, put the baby facing the mirror, hide partially out of view behind the baby, and say, "Where's Mommy? Where did Mommy go?" and then pop out so he can see you in the mirror and say, "Here's Mommy!" You can also partially cover your baby with a small blanket, making sure he can still see, and pretend you cannot see him and say, "Where's baby? Where did he go?" and then, taking the blanket off him, say, "There he is! He was hiding!"

Or try this: Starting slowly, wiggle your fingers, saying, "I've got tickle fingers . . . I've got tickle fingers . . . the tickle fingers are coming to get [baby's name] . . . they are getting closer . . . they got his little knees! They got his little knees!" Then tickle the baby's knees. Repeat with other parts of his body where he likes to be tickled gently. The educational part of the game is having the baby start to anticipate what you're about to do. Even though he's not ready to learn specific words for body parts yet, he'll learn that language can be part of fun social games.

 WHERE'S MOMMY?

Play peekaboo behind the diaper before putting it on. ("Where is Mommy?" will be a favorite game for a long time to come!)

 FUNNY MOMMY!

Make funny faces at the baby while you change her: stick out your tongue, whistle, make your lips vibrate, or make a popping noise with your finger in your mouth. Babies love funny faces and sounds! Reinforce her paying attention to your funny faces by saying, "You like that! Let's do it again!" and making a different funny face.

 SOCK OFF!

Pull the baby's sock most of the way off and see if he can get it the rest of the way off himself. Make a big deal out of celebrating when he does it. If he's interested, but can't pull it off, you can put your hands around his and help him pull it off, then make a big deal: "There it goes! Sock is off!" If he likes this, you can put just the toe on again and help him pull it off again.

Bathtime

 LET'S BLOW BUBBLES

Bathtime is a great time to blow bubbles. Bubbles are a great toy for little ones, because they demonstrate cause and effect and encourage visual tracking. Your baby may think it's very funny to see you pop the bubbles with different parts of your body. For example, you can try to pop one with your nose, kick one with your foot, or clap one between your hands. Each time one pops, say "POP!" and suck in your breath and make a surprised mouth in an O-shape, wowed face. Your baby will enjoy your surprised face and exclamations as much as the bubbles!

 SURPRISE BAGS

Put ordinary household items and small waterproof toys into a bag. Pull out one at a time and hold it near your face and eyes and clearly say its name (e.g., "spoon"). Then let the baby hold it and drop it into the water. As it drops, make a funny sound, like "splash!" or "plunk!" Shrug your shoulders and put your palms facing up and say, "What's next?" Then take the next thing out of the bag. After a couple of items, stop and wait for the baby to signal you to continue by making eye contact, vocalizing, or reaching for the bag. As long as you place different items in the bag each time, this game will never get old!

 BUBBLE BATH

If you put some bubble bath into the bath, it can be great fun to hide things in bubbles. For example, you can give yourself a "bubble beard" and say, "Where is Mommy's chin?" and then wipe the bubbles off your chin and say, "Here's Mommy's chin!" You can cover rubber duckie in bubbles and say, "Where is duckie?" and then wipe off the bubbles and say, "Here he is!" If you have a little mirror, you can put bubbles on your baby's nose, let her see herself, and say, "Where is [baby's name] nose?" and then wipe them off and say, "There it is! There's Baby's nose!" As your baby gets used to this game, she will start to try to wipe the bubbles off herself!

 LINE 'EM UP AND KNOCK 'EM DOWN

If you have child-safe plastic or rubber animals or figures for bathtime, try lining them up on the side of the tub. Each time you put one up, say, "Hello, frog! Hello, duck!" and so on. Then say, "Bye-bye, frog! Bye-bye, duck!" as you knock each one into the bath. As baby gets familiar with this game you can let her (or even help her) be the one to knock them into the bath while you say "Bye-bye." You can then stretch this game out further by saying, "Where is frog? Where did he go?" and then reaching into the bath and saying, "Here he is! Hello, frog!" and putting the frog back on the side of the tub. Then you can repeat this for each animal or character. Eventually when you say, "Where is frog?" your baby will be the one to find it and grab it for you.

 WASHCLOTH GAMES

Play peekaboo behind a washcloth. Bring yourself very close to your baby and slowly pull the washcloth away from your face. If your baby does not begin to reach out and pull it down, you can gently take one of his hands and help him. Take a soapy washcloth and playfully say, "I'm gonna get your arm! I'm gonna get your belly!" while you tickle or gently wipe the body part you named. Try covering animal toys with a washcloth and saying, "All gone! Where did it go?" If your baby doesn't take the washcloth off, you can point to the washcloth and say, "Let's look under here!" or lift the washcloth with a flourish to make the items magically reappear.

Doing Errands/Going for a Walk

 WE'RE GOING FOR A WALK

Continue to carry your child sometimes facing out so she can see the world and sometimes facing you or use a carriage facing you so that you can make eye contact with her often. Point out anything of interest to your child, sharing the experience with her as you walk along.

 "BA" AND "DA"

Your child probably can now discriminate speech sounds (tell them apart) and will be interested in watching your mouth form these different sounds, so as you carry or push him around and stand in lines on errands, sing the alphabet song and also go through and enunciate each sound in the alphabet. Try making up singsong chants such as "apple apple, a, a, a, bubble bottle, ba, ba, ba" or reviving alphabet games from your childhood such as "A, my name is Amy, I live in Alabama, I like to eat apples, and I sell airplanes. A, A, A." Reinforce attention to your mouth by making exaggerated mouth movements that are visually interesting.

 HELP MOMMY SHOP

As you grocery shop, let your child hold any items that are unbreakable and safe to put in her mouth. Sing favorite songs or play music in the car or the market to keep her entertained. A bored baby is a fussy baby.

Chores around the House

 HELP MOMMY COOK

While you're in the kitchen preparing food, let your baby bang spoons on pots and pans, make baby footprints in flour, smell the ingredients, or squish Play-Doh inside a zipper bag.

 FUNNY CLEAN-UP

As you clean up, think about making it into an entertaining show for your baby. Put on some music and incorporate some silly dance moves like standing up on the coffee table or singing into a broom handle.

Playtime

 I CAN SIT!

Give your baby lots of opportunities to strengthen his new physical skills by helping him sit and positioning him to play on both his stomach and his back. Here is an idea to help him strengthen his neck muscles: Place your baby on his tummy and sing one of his favorite songs as you move around the room. This will encourage him to track you visually and to turn his head and neck to do so. If your baby stops looking at you or tracking you, pause your singing. If he does not signal or communicate to you to continue in some way, get down on the floor and regain his attention with eye contact and proximity (and perhaps a new song) and try again.

 I CAN REACH AND ROLL

Try placing toys slightly out of your baby's reach. She will either practice reaching and grasping (raking things toward herself) or signal to you to bring them closer. Place her facing up on a small blanket and gently pick up one side and then the other—you're not trying to roll her all the way over, but rather just rolling her a bit from one side to the other, to give her the experience of feeling her body in different positions. Another rolling game is to place very different interesting-looking objects on each side and roll her from one side to the other, changing her view.

 REAL-WORLD TOYS

Provide a variety of age-appropriate toys (like teethers) and household objects—like a spatula (with no sharp edges) or an empty plastic food container with a lid—to explore by banging, sucking, and touching. Avoid electronic toys that have fast-moving lights and sounds. At this age it's important that your baby learn how the real world works; electronics, which will surely capture his attention, may prevent him from paying attention to real objects and people.

 PEEKABOO AND HIDE AND SEEK

There are many variations on peekaboo and hide and seek, all of which can help your baby understand that when things leave her sight they still exist. Here are some possibilities: Try hiding toys, such as favorite stuffed animals, partly out of view, such as half under a blanket or a pillow. Shrug your shoulders and place your palms facing up, saying, "Where did it go?" You can cover your eyes as if blocking the sun to look a far distance and say, "I don't see it anywhere. Where could it be?" Really exaggerate the puzzled look on your face and keep the pretense going until the baby pulls the toy out. Then celebrate her discovery with enthusiasm: "There it is! Yay! You found it! You're so good at finding things!" You can make the hiding places farther away and make more of the toy hidden as she gets better at this game. If she doesn't uncover the toy, you can prompt her by gently taking her hand and helping her pull the blanket off, saying, "There it is! You found it!"

You can play the same game by partly hiding yourself under a blanket or behind a pillow in reach of where your baby can grab it and reveal you. You can also play this type of game with a music box or any kind of toy that makes continuous sounds. The sounds can act as a cue to help your baby find the missing object.

 ## I DO, YOU DO!

Imitation is a fundamental concept for your baby to learn, and it will help him learn many things in the future. Play a game where you imitate everything the baby does. For example, if he leans to the side, you lean to the side; if he bangs a coaster, you bang a coaster; if he says "ga-ga," you say "ga-ga"; and if he sucks on a toy, you take a turn sucking on a toy. Of course, do this only for a few minutes and make it clear it's a funny game. As soon as he stops enjoying this, go on to something else.

 ## I CAN MOVE THINGS

Help your baby get some practice with fine motor skills with some of these games: Set out some muffin tins in front of the baby and help her throw a ball and see where it goes (usually it will roll a bit on top and land in one of the muffin holes). Hold toys just out of her reach. Be patient while she figures out how to swat them. Hold things that make noise (like a drum) just within reach of her feet and hold them still while she figures out how to kick them. Alternatively, hold your hands up and make a funny sound (like "pow") each time she kicks a hand.

 ## FAMILY ALBUM

Show your baby a photo album of family and friends. Make a page for each person. Sometimes you can go through it quickly, just saying every person's name, and sometimes you can go through it slowly by talking to the baby about each person. They now make recordable photo albums. If you can get friends and family to record a message, you can play the sound of their voices on each page for your baby. If she shows no interest in family faces and voices after you've showed these to her a few times, try putting it away for a couple of months and then bringing it out to try again.

 ## PINWHEEL

Babies like to watch things spin. You can turn this into an opportunity for back-and-forth play by blowing on a pinwheel and making it go and then pausing and waiting for your baby to signal to you with his eye contact or his body that he wants you to do it again. Then say, "Spin? Okay!" or other similar, simple words. You can also say, "Ready, set, go!" as you help him spin it on the word "go!"

TROT-TROT TO BOSTON

Sit the baby on your knees, holding her securely, and bounce her up and down while saying, "Trot Trot to Boston, Trot Trot to Lynn, Watch out little [baby's name] so you don't fall in!" (On the word "in," give your baby a little dip.) "Trot trot to Boston, Trot trot to town, watch out little [baby's name] so you don't fall down!" (On the word "down," give him a little dip.)

 BOUNCE TIME

Hold your baby in a standing position facing you so that his legs are supporting a bit of weight beneath him and help him bounce up and down while singing "The Tigger Song" (look for it on YouTube or pick any song that you can put "bouncing" in). This is good both for exercise and for practicing eye contact. This can be particularly fun on a large ball. If your baby likes this a lot, try pausing when he looks away and waiting for eye contact, a babbling sound, a rocking or bouncing movement, or any other attempt to communicate that he wants more before resuming the bouncing and singing.

 WAY UP HIGH

You can "fly" the baby up high in your arms, saying, "Way up high!" and then bring her down, saying, "Way down low!" Try changing the pitch of your voice so that you say "Way up high" in a high-pitched voice and "Way down low," in a low, deep voice. You can also sing "The Grand Old Duke of York, he has ten thousand men, he marched them *up* [as you fly the baby up] to the top of the hill, and he marched them *down* again [as you bring the baby down], and when they were *up* they were *up* [as you fly the baby up again], and when they were *down* they were *down* [as you bring the baby down], and when they were only halfway up [baby up] they were neither *up* nor *down* [down]." Be sure to emphasize the key words "up" and "down" as you repeat the chant. Another variation is to hold the baby while you move up or down by stepping up on a bottom stair and then stepping down to the floor again. Help your baby fly like an airplane by supporting her chest and belly with one or both of your arms. Most babies like this, but some will find it scary; if she's one of these, move on to something else.

 HELIUM BALLOON

Holding the balloon string together, you can say, "Ready, set, go!" and let the balloon go together on the word "go" and watch it fly up to the ceiling. Say, "Way up high!" Then reel it in together and say, "Way down low." (When the baby gets older, you'll be able to expand on this game by saying, "Ready, set . . . ," and then waiting for him to make a sound or movement with his body that lets you know he wants you to let it go or pull it back down.)

DISGUISE FACE

Draw extra attention to your face by placing stickers, a clown nose, nonscary Halloween masks, or oversized plastic glasses on your face (anything that your baby can safely pull off). The baby will find it a fun game to pull these things off and watch you put them back on.

 SONGS FOR MOVING HANDS

Babies love hearing sounds and music while watching your hands move. Try these tried-and-true songs: "I'm a Little Teapot," "The Itsy Bitsy Spider," "The Wheels on the Bus," "If You're Happy and You Know It." A variation of these finger plays is to make motions directly on your baby's body—for example, making her legs go around in a bicycle motion as you sing "The wheels on the bus go round and round," making your finger crawl up her body as you sing "The itsy bitsy spider crawled up the water spout."

And here are some rhymes with hand motions:

- "Two little apples up in a tree (hold fists up in the air), I shook that tree as hard as I *could* (pretend to shake a tree). Boom! Went the apple (bring one fist to the floor), Boom! Went the apple (bring the other fist to the floor)." Make munching noises as you bring one fist (apple) to your mouth and then the other: "Mmmm-mmmmm *good*!"

- "I'm a little bunny with two bunny ears (make bunny ears), I really love to hop hop hop (hop three times). I'm so tired! I'm so tired! (yawn and stretch) Now it's time to stop." (Lie down and pretend to fall asleep.)

- "Here is the church (interlock hands so that fingers are inside), here is the steeple (raise two index fingers to a point touching each other above the interlocked hands), open up the doors (open your thumbs), and look at all the people (turn over your hands and wiggle your fingers)."

CHAPTER 15

6–9 Months

Your baby is really becoming a little person. He is much more interested in the world around him; when he starts to crawl, he will be exploring all over the place! His temperament and personality may be emerging, and he is ready to interact actively with other people.

WHAT 6- TO 9-MONTH-OLDS ARE LEARNING

Social Skills: Imitation, Turn Taking, and Sharing

Your 6- to 9-month-old baby is becoming a much more social creature and will be fascinated by imitation and eager to learn early social "rules" such as turn taking and sharing. This is a great age to get down on the floor and model the kinds of movement and play in which you want your baby to engage. She'll be intrigued by the idea of doing what you do and can learn from imitation.

Eye contact is usually the first way babies can "take turns" in communication—making eye contact with you tells you they want to continue the interaction, whereas breaking eye contact tells you they want to discontinue. In other words, if you're pushing your baby gently on a baby swing, tickling her, or feeding her, you could pause and wait for her to look at you or make sounds to request more before each push or tickle or bite. Even if your child doesn't yet understand your words, she'll start to understand that you're waiting for her to respond or communicate with you in some way before continuing the interaction. When she makes eye contact, say something like, "More swing? Okay! Here we go!" or "More cereal? Yummy!" and continue. The idea is to teach your child to pay attention to you during play and begin to "take turns" communicating with you.

You can also teach and encourage sharing at this age by making a big deal out of it when your baby tries to share her peas or drool-soaked cracker with you ("My turn? Thank you!") and also by asking her to share her toys with you by putting out your hand for her to give you things and, if she does not, by gently taking them, taking a quick turn, and then handing them back.

Making Intentional Sounds and Gestures to Refer to People and Things

Most babies begin to babble and develop the precursors of language before they begin to speak. These sounds consist of exclamations ("Doo-ick!" "Ba!"), gestures (reaching, shaking head), and babbling that has the melody of the language the baby has been hearing. For example, your baby might say "Ba ba ba? Ba ba!" using a rising intonation, as if asking a question, followed by another that sounds more like an exclamation. Your baby will begin to make associations between your words and actions and their meanings—for example, that clapping means you're happy and that a head shake means "no."

Research has shown that there are a few ways that parents can help their children learn language:

1. *Make sure your baby hears lots and lots of words.* You want your baby to hear complex sentences so he can hear lots of sounds and hear the way grammar and tone fit together, which is why reading books and narrating what is happening around you is good for him. At the same time, you want to give him lots of practice and repetition with hearing simple words. In other words, during this first year, make sure there are plenty of times during the day when you're using one word at a time to communicate; for example, you could say, "Up? Okay! Up!" and then pick your baby up.

2. *Label the focus of your child's attention.* For example, if your baby is looking back and forth between you and his dad, you might say "Mama" when he looks at Mama and "Dada" when he looks at Dad, pointing to each of you in turn. Young children don't understand that your attention may be focused on something different from their own, so if they're looking intently at a bird or a balloon, label the object *they* are focused on and share the enjoyment of that object of interest by sharing a smile or making a simple comment about it before attempting to draw their attention to something else.

3. *Respond to your child's actions as if they were meaningful.* We talked earlier about the importance of making your actions and words *contingent* on your child's actions and words. **Contingent responding is the single most influential thing you can do to help your child learn language.** So even if you're not sure whether your child just said a word or simply made a nonsense sound, or pointed to some

object of interest versus only reaching for it, respond as if it was a word or a meaningful gesture ("Yes! Happy! Daddy *is* happy! He's laughing" or "Oh, you want a banana! Okay, here you go!"). You will be teaching your child that all of his behavior is meaningful in the social world.

4. *Incorporate gestures into your language as much as you can.* Many children who are slow to learn to talk will learn faster if they're taught to use some simple gestures and signs. You can even make up your own signs and gestures to go with words, as long as you're consistent. You may find that your child can communicate with you by making his hands shape a ball or swing back and forth like a swing before he can say the word "swing" or "ball."

In addition to using lots of gestures, you can start to teach your baby to follow a point by touching and tapping the thing you're pointing to so that it makes a sound as you point or try to draw his attention by doing something funny or interesting. Using his name as you draw his attention to things, and then waiting for eye contact to share a smile, or before showing him what an object does or how it works, will help him get into the habit of checking back with you regularly. You want your child to learn that you really have something worthwhile to show him when you call his name or point to something and say, "Look!" So make sure you're calling his attention to something interesting as often as you can (a cool toy, a yummy food, or a fun thing you're about to do like swoop in for belly kisses).

Expressing Emotion and Affection

Between 6 and 9 months, infants should begin to display a wider range of facial expressions and begin to demonstrate their affection for you in different ways (for example, giving your cheek an open-mouthed gummy kiss). You can encourage this by exaggerating your own facial expressions and mirroring your infant's facial expression. For example, you might imitate her sad face and say, "I'm sad! I don't want to leave Grandpa's house!" before soothing her. You may also want to start bringing more emotional themes into your play. A puppet you play with can be grouchy because he is tired or because he hates to eat peas. When you play a simple form of hide and seek (for example, by holding up a washcloth or towel in front of your baby's face for a few seconds and pretending you can't find her), you may want to really exaggerate your expression of surprise when you find her. You want to encourage your baby to express as much positive emotion as possible, so return often to the games, songs, books, and other activities that make her smile and laugh. However, babies cannot be happy all the time; they will also be cranky, scared, frustrated, and sad at times. So aim to maximize the positive emotions, but be prepared to *acknowledge*, imitate, and give language to the negative emotions, too, and then show the baby that you will help him deal with his negative emotions.

Try to acknowledge the baby's emotions whenever you can. If she looks sad, for example, you can make an exaggerated sad face and say, "You feel sad." Then you could see if a cuddle will comfort her. When your child drops her doll on the floor, you can pretend to talk for the doll and say, "Ouch, that hurt! I fell down and got a boo-boo!" When you're playing with a jack-in-the-box, you can make a scared face and say, "We feel nervous!" Or open your eyes wide, eyebrows raised, and say, "We feel excited," and when the jack pops out make an exaggerated surprised face. Most babies will enjoy being mildly startled, especially if you make a surprised face and then laugh. If your child is distressed by this level of surprise, and cries when startled, you can tone it down by moving the jack-in-the-box farther away from her or by preparing your child just before the jack-in-the-box pops up ("Here he comes!") or substitute a pop-up toy that you can control (like a pop-up puppet), so you can make it pop up more slowly.

When your child is happy or laughing, say, "You're so happy about_____," and take her hands and jump up and down with her to show her that you can be happy together. When she laughs, say, "You're being silly!" and tickle her so that she sees that laughing with you is better than laughing by herself. Remember, you want to stretch out her expression of positive emotions and teach her to share her emotions with you. You also want to react with visible emotion to the things she does in order to help her learn the impact of her behavior on others. So if she sticks a toy in her mouth, you could say, "That's yucky!" or "That's silly! You don't EAT telephones; you TALK on telephones!" (**Note: You should not react this way to something you don't want the child to do again, such as sticking a toy that she could choke on in her mouth.** Remember, the behaviors you pay a lot of special attention to are likely to happen more often in the future.)

It's also a good idea to begin to teach your child how to soothe herself when she's upset. For example, if your child is fussy, you could say, "Let's go find your teddy bear and blankie. They always make you feel better. You keep them in your bed." As you say this you can be guiding her (if she's crawling) or carrying her to the place where she keeps these special objects.

Playing with Toys

By 6 months, babies are ready to be introduced to the world of toys. The best types of toys are cause-and-effect toys (push a button and it makes a sound) and toys that encourage fine motor development, such as stacking rings, blocks, and nesting cups. In contrast, some of the hardest toys to create shared attention with are toys with lights, sounds, and music. You may want to put away these types of electronic toys during your playtime unless you can find a way to make yourself more interesting than the toy. For example, if your child likes a toy where he presses a button and music plays, you can sing the same tune and do a silly dance, or play along with a percussion instrument like a triangle, a child's tambourine, or a maraca. You may find that he starts to press the button and then looks at you expectantly, and maybe he'll even want a turn with the instrument.

When you play with your baby, try to position yourself face to face and try to hold some of the desired items, such as the rings or blocks, so that when he wants to continue playing, he must look at you or interact with you to get the next piece of the toy.

Creeping and Crawling

Your baby will be very interested in mastering different kinds of movement that help her get to what she wants. This ability to develop a plan and carry it out will help her begin to develop a sense of being able to do things for herself. Games that help encourage her to practice moving her body, such as making a Cheerios trail for her to follow, giving her a balloon to try to grab and then scoot after when it gets away (if you will be watching her at all times, since balloons are a choking hazard), placing a different toy on each step of the stairs, or making a tunnel for her to crawl through, are wonderful at this age. One word of caution, however: A baby must be developmentally ready for crawling or scooting on her behind. If she's not ready, pushing her to do these things will be not only useless but upsetting to her, as will setting up temptations (like chasing the balloon). If you see that she is trying to move but isn't ready, back off and try again in a month.

Object Permanence

Your baby is beginning to get a grasp on object permanence—the idea that an object or person exists even when it is not visible. This development makes peekaboo and hiding games essential parts of your play and teaching activities at this age.

Eating

Babies are generally ready to begin eating solid foods by 6 months. Ask your pediatrician when your baby is ready. This gives you an exciting opportunity to help establish variety in your baby's diet right from the beginning and to share in the excitement of introducing new foods. It also means you'll begin to have mealtimes where you are sitting face to face, which will allow for play and teaching sessions right from the high chair.

THINGS TO WATCH FOR

Each child develops at her own pace, but talk to your baby's doctor if your 6- to 9-month-old

- does not show joyful expressions.
- does not smile back at you when you smile.
- does not respond to loud noises.
- does not show interest in faces.
- turns away when you make eye contact.
- stiffens and cries when held by familiar caregivers.
- cannot hold her head up or sit upright without assistance.
- is not babbling with both consonant and vowels sounds by 7 months.

HOW YOU CAN HELP
YOUR 6- TO 9-MONTH-OLD LEARN

Following are some ideas for helping your baby learn all the new skills he is mastering at this age. As always, use the ones that seem most interesting to your baby, and of course you should feel free to think up your own games and activities.

Here are some general principles:

- Continue the activities from previous sections that have been working for you and your baby.
- Treat all communication as intentional.
- Begin to coordinate shared attention between you and your baby toward an object (for example, toys).
- Introduce sharing and turn taking.
- Make ample use of gestures, including beginning to point to exciting things, nodding and shaking your head, and perhaps learning some baby "signs." We'll suggest some in this book (see Chapter 17), but the Internet is a good source for baby sign language as well.
- Use repetitive language and "motherese" (exaggerate vowel sounds and the ups and downs of your sentences).
- Learn to make yourself the center of your child's happy attention—this requires learning to make your behavior contingent on his, as discussed earlier:
  o Reinforce behavior you want to see, such as attempts at communication (with praise and smiles and tickles and attention).
  o Play eye contact games like using the baby looking at you as a trigger for pushing him in a baby swing.
  o Remain in charge of desired items (food, toys) so he will look at you to get what he wants.
  o Place yourself strategically in front of him to make it easy for him to look at you and try to be the most fun/interesting thing in the room.

Waking Up/Bedtime Routines (Including Story Time)

 WAKE UP, BABY!

Try stretching out morning greetings as much as possible. So not only should you greet your baby with an enthusiastic "Good morning!" but also try greeting all of his stuffed animals ("Good morning, teddy!"), lifting up the curtains or shades and saying, "Good morning, day!" and perhaps even pictures of various family members ("Good morning, Auntie!" "Good morning, Grandma!").

SLEEPY TIME

Kiss all family members and stuffed animals good night, saying, "Kiss brother, good night, brother," "Kiss teddy, good night, teddy." Go around the house and turn out the lights together (you can help your baby flip the switch), saying, "Now it's dark—good night, kitchen! Now it's dark—good night, bathroom!" After you turn the lights off in your baby's room, you can hold a flashlight together and shine it on different items in the room, saying, "Good night, crib, good night, closet," and so on.

 LET'S READ A BOOK

Not only does reading books to your baby stimulate language and cognitive development, but research has shown that reading in a specific way enhances these benefits even further. Rather than just reading the words exactly as they are written (although this is also fun and important), try sometimes creating a back-and-forth dialogue around the story with your baby. Of course, at this age you will need to supply both sides of the dialogue, such as, "Who's that? It's Goldilocks! Oh no! Look, baby bear feels sad! Uh-oh! Goldilocks looks scared! What is she going to do next? Oh look, she is running away!" As you say words from the story, point to them in the picture. For example, if you're reading *Goodnight, Moon* point to the spoon as you say "spoon" and to the mittens as you say "mittens." This provides your child with an extra cue for matching the sounds of words with their pictures. Babies at this age especially love "lift the flap" books, which allow them to play peekaboo with their favorite pictures and enhance their memory skills. Babies at this age also tend to love textured books such as *Pat the Bunny* that allow them to reach out and feel different textures (such as a bunny's soft fur or a daddy's scratchy beard).

Feeding Time

 YUMMY/YUCKY

When your baby first begins eating, give her one bite at a time and watch her face. If she grimaces or pushes it away, say, "Eww, yucky!" If she looks happy and reaches for more, say, "Mmmm. Yummy!" When she makes eye contact or reaches for more, say something like, "More _____?" (naming the food). If she reaches but does not make eye contact, try holding the next bite of food up to your face so that she "has" to make eye contact.

 HERE COMES THE PLANE

Make eating playful when you spoon-feed your baby by pretending that the spoon is an airplane flying around before coming in for a landing or a chirping bird looking for a place to perch. Another silly game is to hold out a bite of food and pretend to cover or close your eyes, saying, "I'm gonna catch a little [baby's favorite animal]," and then when the baby takes a bite uncover your eyes and look surprised: "Oh the [animal] must have gotten away! Let's try again!"

 FEED MOMMY?

You can lean forward and open your mouth and say, "Feed Mommy?" If your baby puts a piece of the food in your mouth, say, "Thank you for sharing! Mommy is so happy!" or just "Thank you." You can bring over various dolls or stuffed animals that you don't mind getting a little crumby and say, "Feed horsie?" and so on. You can also make the doll pretend to think various foods are "yummy" or "yucky."

 WHERE DID IT GO?

Try tying different lightweight toys to string or ribbon and tie the other end of the string or ribbon to the high chair. Let the baby knock them off of his high chair and then reel them back in (you will have to teach him how to do this, but he'll get it with practice). Your baby will love to compare the sound of something like keys hitting the floor with something rubber hitting the floor and will enjoy seeing things "disappear" and "reappear." Using "tools" (in this case, the string to reel in the toy) strengthens cognitive and motor development.

Diaper Changing and Dressing

 PEEKABOO!

Put a towel or cloth over your head and say, "Peeka . . ." while leaning closer until baby yanks the cloth off—as soon as she does, say "Boo!" and laugh. Soon she'll understand her part in this game.

 DRESSING SONG

Pick a simple tune to sing (for example, "jammies, jammies, off, off, off") or change the words to a song you know (Cookie monster's "C Is for Cookie" song could become the "D Is for Diaper" song) and make it a routine part of dressing or diaper changing. If your baby likes this song, you can start singing it, and when he looks away, pause and wait for eye contact before you continue singing it.

 LOOK AT MAMA!

As long as you're changing the baby, play silly games that involve your face and create anticipation. For example, puff your cheeks up and then gently bring your baby's hands to your cheeks as if he is "squishing" out the air. You can make him really squish your cheeks to blow out all the air at once, or you can make him give your cheeks tiny quick taps, each one letting out a small burst of air from your mouth. You can blow on his face, his belly, and so forth. Then you can use his feet to squish the air out of your puffed-up cheeks and you can blow on his feet. Reinforce eye contact by pausing and waiting for eye contact before you continue the game.

 YUMMY BABY!

Put your mouth behind your shirt or make your hands into circles around your eyes (something to create a visual cue to your baby that the game has started) and say playfully, perhaps in a silly Cookie Monster–like voice, "I am the baby monster. I am going to get the baby's fingers and gobble them up. Mmm, delicious! I am going to get the baby's toes and gobble them up! Mmm, delicious!" If your baby enjoys this game, give him the visual signal you've created and then wait for eye contact before you start the game.

Bathtime

 RAINBOW BATHTIME

Use color tablets; hold out two different-color bath tablets and let your baby choose which one to "Drop! Splash!" into the water. You can watch it dissolve and let the baby "stir" the water with a spoon and watch the whole bath change color (again while using simple, singsong words like "Mix, mix, mix in the bath, bath, bath!").

 DRAWING IN THE TUB

With foaming soap or shaving cream or bathtub crayons, draw or squirt different shapes on the wall. After labeling them, let your baby wash them away with a squirt bottle and a washcloth. Sing the "Clean Up" song as she washes. You can try this with letters as well—draw soapy letters on the bathtub wall one at a time and practice playing with the sounds. You can show your baby your mouth (and even let her feel it) as you exaggerate "Ahhh, Aaaah, Aaaaah," and "Baaa, baaa, baaa," and so on through the alphabet, pausing to give her a turn for the sounds she is willing to try. Give her lots of praise when she gives it a try. Of course, she is still too young to learn the letters, but it's a great time to introduce the idea of imitating specific sounds.

 LET'S GO FISHING

Fishing games can be great fun in the bath for years to come. Get your baby some toy fish, or cut some up from aluminum foil or sheets of colored foam that you can buy at a craft store. Use these along with a net with a handle. Use the same language you use during tickle games, such as, "I'm gonna get you . . . I got you!" as you try to catch fish in the net. When he's ready, help your baby go fishing with hand-over-hand help and let him try it for himself when he wants to.

 FILL AND SPILL

This game teaches your baby to fill and empty containers. It is as simple as getting various shapes and sizes of containers and teaching her how to fill them with water by holding them under the faucet or submerging them in the bath water. As your baby does this, say, "Fill . . . ," (with a rising intonation) and then show her how to dump them out, saying, "Spill!" Waterwheels are also a lot of fun at bathtime. Show your baby how to pour the water onto the waterwheel to make it spin—a great lesson in cause and effect.

 POP THE BUBBLE

Your baby has been enjoying tracking bubbles visually as you blow them in the bath. Now you can give him a chance to pop them himself by blowing a bubble, catching it on the wand, and holding it next to his hand. Say, "Pop!" when he pops it. After a couple of bubbles, you can hold the wand near your face and wait for eye contact before you let him pop the bubble.

 SILLY ICE CUBES

As long as the weather and the bath water are warm, try making "silly" ice cubes. For example, take different-shaped plastic containers. Hide a small toy or action figure inside, fill them with water, add a few drops of food coloring, and then freeze them overnight. When you let your baby take a bath with a silly ice cube, she will have fun touching it ("Cold!"), trying to grab it ("Slippery! Oops, it got away!"), watching it melt ("It's getting smaller and smaller!"), and finally rescuing the small toy figure from inside it ("You got it!"). As with all small objects, be on guard for your baby popping it in his mouth.

Doing Errands/Going for a Walk

 BABY SIGNS

Look at Chapter 17 for pictures of a few baby signs for simple words for things you tend to see on your walks together and check the Internet for others that you encounter frequently. You can also make up your own signs, as long as you use the same ones consistently. Not only can you point these things out verbally to your child, but the matching visual input also will help your baby learn the word faster. It may even help her learn to communicate the word faster. For example, babies can often sniff (the sign for "flower") before they can articulate the word "flower."

Chores around the House

 LAUNDRY TIME

You can sit your baby on top of or next to the washing machine, or hold him, as you hand him the dirty clothes to put in. Of course, if he's sitting, keep a hand on him, even if he can sit by himself, or put him in a baby seat where he can reach the opening of the washing machine. Every time he puts something in, you can say, "In!" or you can label the clothes: "In you go, blue shirt!" or "Rainbow socks in!" After a couple of articles of clothing, pause and wait for eye contact before you hand your baby the next piece. If you need to, prompt eye contact by holding a colorful item of clothing near your face.

 BABY HELPING MOMMY COOK

When you're cooking, give your baby a pot and a spoon to play with. She'll probably just use them to make noise, but this can be the beginning of her "helping" you in the kitchen.

Playtime

 ANIMAL TICKLES OR KISSES

Place your baby securely on one side of the room and go to the other side. Say, "Froggy tickles!" and hop over to your baby saying, "Ribbit!" until you can reach him and tickle him. Say, "Duckie tickles!" and waddle over, saying, "Quack!" until you reach him and tickle him. Say, "Butterfly kisses!" and flap your wings as you fly over to him and give him a butterfly kiss on his cheek. You can crawl like a bug, fly like an eagle, slither like a snail, and so on. You're teaching your child about animal sounds and movements as you play. (When he's older, he may enjoy calling out what kind of animal tickles you should offer next.) If the baby is enjoying the game, pause and wait for eye contact before you do the next animal or just before you swoop in for the tickle or kiss.

 AHHHHHHHHHH BOOM!

Babies of this age still love simple anticipation games. For example, lean your head backward and then make it come slowly forward toward your baby's, saying, "Ahh-hhhhhhhh . . ." And then touch your heads together saying, "Boom!"

 VEHICLE RIDES

Give your baby an airplane ride by holding her firmly on top of a pillow. You make the airplane pillow go down the runway faster and faster and then lift off into the sky and fly around the room. You can turn a laundry basket into a boat or choo-choo train by shouting "All aboard!" and making "chugga choo choo" sounds as you push the baby around, or by placing the laundry basket on top of a blue blanket and pretending to make the boat rock in the waves. (Singing a train or boat song as you go can be fun too!) Don't go too fast or too high, especially if it's scary to the child, and always make sure your child is secure; if your laundry basket is tippy, keep one hand on it.

 NOW IT'S . . . (BIG/SMALL, LONG/SHORT, OPEN/SHUT, ETC.)

Babies love watching things change form, and they are actively learning cause and effect. Finding a toy (such as a balloon or stretchy tube or a collapsing ball) that gets bigger or smaller or longer or shorter can be fascinating. Even something like an umbrella that looks dramatically different open and shut is great. Keep your language simple, like, "Now it's little . . . now it's big!" In a few months you might be able to say, "Now it's . . . ," and wait for your baby to fill in the blank! As with other games, if he's enjoying the open and close, after a couple of turns, wait for eye contact before you do it again.

 TOUCH AND FEEL BOX

You can either purchase one or make your own by emptying an oatmeal canister and placing a cut-off pantyhose or knee-high section over the top or cutting small holes in the top of a shoebox. The important part of this game is that the baby can feel inside the box but not see. This will strengthen her sense of touch. You can fill this box with different items each day. Use simple words such as "I feel . . ." when you and baby are reaching inside and "I see . . ." when you pull out items. Or "What is it?" when she reaches inside and "Oh, it's a ball!" when she pulls it out.

 PAPER TOWEL ROLL GAMES

An empty paper towel or wrapping paper roll can be perfect for object permanence games. Show your baby how you can send cars and balls through and they come out the other side with simple words like "Bye-bye, car! Hello, car!" You can also stuff tissues and silky scarves inside and then let the baby pull them out. Magic! Be very enthusiastic when he pulls the item out and then wait for eye contact before putting another object in. If necessary, put your face where he can easily see you or wiggle the scarf or tissue near your face. When you get eye contact, say something like "Great! Let's do it again!" and put the next thing inside. (As long as you've got the paper towel roll out, try talking into it to see if your baby finds your voice funny when you do this.)

 MUSIC MAKER

If you have child-safe musical instruments to let your child explore, great. If not, take a few small plastic or other child-safe containers and fill them with different things: rice, dry beans, coins, jingle bells. Empty plastic water bottles with screw tops work especially well for this. Let your child play by shaking each one to hear the different sounds. Try saying and modeling different simple rhymes with this game, such as, "Shake it to the left. Shake it to the right. SHAKE IT REALLY FAST WITH ALL YOUR MIGHT!" or "Shake it FAST. Shake it SLOW. Shake it up high. And shake it down LOW!" You can practice taking turns, shaking it, waiting for eye contact, and then handing it to baby, helping her shake it if needed.

 PLAY BALL!

There are lots of things you can do with balls. For example, gather balls of all different sizes. Multiple examples of a ball will teach your child to pay attention to an object's shape and function rather than properties such as color. In addition, he'll enjoy observing the different ways different balls roll. Sit facing each other with your legs open and roll the ball back and forth for your first game of catch. Take balls and also cylinders (empty plastic cartons or cups, empty cylindrical containers for oatmeal, baking soda, raisins, etc.) and also household objects of other shapes. Take each object one at a time and try to roll it on the floor. When it rolls, say, "Rolls!" When it doesn't, say, "Oops! Doesn't roll!" This will be one of your baby's first science experiments! Or set up empty plastic soda bottles or anything lightweight a few feet from where you and baby are sitting and then take turns rolling the balls into the empty bottles to "knock 'em down!" Since you'll be facing each other, this is a great game for waiting for eye contact, helping your baby if necessary by wiggling the ball in front of your face. You could also say, "One, two, THREE," and roll the ball on the count of three. After he has learned this, you could say, "One, two . . . ," then pause and wait for eye contact before saying, "THREE!" and rolling the ball.

 LET'S MOVE

Sometimes encouraging crawling is as simple as giving your baby something to chase after. For example, you can place a ball, or a rolling toy on wheels, just past her reach and let her crawl to it and touch it. When she touches it, she may push it away, and she'll need to crawl more to catch up. Similarly, you can tape different magazine pictures to an empty oatmeal container. Your baby will be interested in seeing the different pictures roll away as she tries to grab it, and she'll be motivated to chase after it. Make a tunnel. Babies enjoy scooting and crawling through tunnels. You can keep placing yourself in front of your baby with your legs apart to be a "Mommy tunnel," or you can make tunnels by setting two chairs next to each other with a blanket on top, or folding a large play mat, or opening two ends of a large cardboard box. A bunch of different tunnels together, with a pillow mountain thrown in, can make a great crawling obstacle course. One thing to remember is that babies are physically ready to crawl at different ages; pushing your baby to do something, like crawl or, later, walk, when she's not ready will only frustrate both of you. You might want to check with your pediatrician if you're not sure whether your baby is ready.

WHERE'S BABY?

A silly game is to pretend that you can't see your baby. Pretend to look in the other directions, under the couch, or out the window as you say, "Where is _____? Where did he go?" before your eyes land on him and you say, "There you are!" with big smiles and kisses. A variation of this is to take a stuffed animal or toy and cover it partially with a blanket and say, "Where is _____?" or "Where did it go?" Once your baby gets good at this, try covering it all the way up, hiding it behind your back, under your shirt, or inside your hands.

 POP-UP TIME

A popular type of toy is one that involves turning a crank or pushing a button to get animals or characters to "pop up" or "pop out" from underneath or behind a closed door. Usually the first thing babies can do is to close the doors. You can play a turn-taking game by opening the doors and greeting the animals ("Hello, giraffe! Hello, panda!") and then let your baby close the doors as you say, "Good-bye, giraffe! Good-bye, panda!" You and your baby can together make a big deal of waving good-bye to the animals and even blowing them kisses. Then make an exaggerated gesture with your palms up and say, "Where did they go?" You can stretch this game out by looking around for the animals or shaking the toy or knocking on its doors, or you can get right back to opening the doors and greeting the animals. As your baby's fine motor skills develop, help her learn to open the doors or press the pop-up levers herself so she gets a chance to play both sides of the game.

 FIND THE NOISE

Find any toy or object that makes continuous sound—a music player, a ticking clock, and so on. Hide the toy out of sight and then teach the baby to follow the sound to find it. Start with easy hiding spots (for example, place it under a blanket right in front of him) and then make it progressively more challenging.

 WHERE IS THUMBKIN?

Sing the song "Where Is Thumbkin?" giving each hand a very different voice (your left hand could sing in a high voice and your right hand in a deep, low voice). Once your baby has learned how the song goes, you could pause and wait for eye contact or a gesture that she wants you to continue and then finish the song.

 MIRROR PLAY

Mirror play is also a great way to encourage eye contact in very young children (and it encourages self-awareness!). Some children find it easier to make eye contact in a mirror than face to face. If this is so for your child, you might think of more games to do in the mirror and take lots of opportunities to make and reward eye contact with enthusiastic praise. You can encourage eye contact and facial imitation while sitting with your child on your lap in front of the mirror and making funny faces and funny sounds, like animal noises, or sneezes or coughs or hiccups. You might take a washable marker and draw shapes on the mirror and encourage your child to scribble on it with his marker. You can also practice making different emotional expressions. There are a number of books that show babies making emotional or silly faces, and you can try to copy these expressions in the mirror. Or you could practice making different movements like raising your arms in the air or putting your hands on your head. You can give silly rewards like putting stickers on your faces and then looking in the mirror every time your child does a good imitation, as well as praise and a cuddle.

Babies and toddlers love to watch their appearance change in the mirror, so try keeping a basket of silly hats and maybe a clown wig next to the mirror and playing a game of trying them on and taking them off one another. (Remember, we always want to put a lot of emotion into these games, so every time your child takes off his hat you can say, for example, "You took off your hat, hooray!" and clap your hands and cheer.) Babies also enjoy watching you "sneak up on them" in the mirror and tickle or kiss them from behind. You could blow bubbles toward the mirror and watch them pop on it.

CHAPTER 16

9–12 Months

By 9–12 months most babies are getting really mobile, scooting on their behind, crawling on all fours, or crawling on elbows and pushing off with their legs. Of course, they have no sense of danger as they indulge their curiosity about the world, so now's the time to childproof the house, if you haven't already. They are exploring with their hands and their mouths and interacting with other people, including paying a lot of attention to others' speech.

WHAT 9- TO 12-MONTH-OLDS ARE LEARNING

Making More Intentional Sounds and Gestures to Communicate

Between 9 and 12 months your baby should begin to show you that he recognizes the meaning of more of your words. For example, he should begin to respond to hearing you say "No!" by pausing (although usually not for more than a second or two!), and he should regularly turn his head when you call his name. He should recognize (if not produce) the words "mama" and "dada," turning to look toward Mom and Dad (or other caregivers) when he hears their names. By 12 months your baby should be able to follow a simple instruction such as "Wave good-bye" and "Give me a kiss." Between 9 and 12 months your baby should also begin to use more body language to communicate with you. For example, he should begin to clap when he is pleased or thinks you are pleased and to shake his head "no" when you offer him foods he does not want. He should begin to hold up toys that he wants you to see because he is enjoying them and wants you to share in his enjoyment. He should also show you affection, with hugs or nuzzles, or pats or (sloppy) kisses. His sounds should become more recognizable, and you may hear him beginning to try to imitate your words, especially common first words such as "mama," "dada," and "baba." He should be using a pointing finger to show you something interesting or something he wants, although he may only be able to point to things that are close by.

Developing a Sense of Humor

Babies begin to develop their sense of humor between 6 and 12 months. For example, although 6-month-old babies will look longer toward absurd events than typical events, they will laugh only if their caregiver is also laughing. By 1 year old, most babies laugh at absurd events even if their caregiver is not laughing. You can encourage the development of your baby's sense of humor by purposely acting silly and laughing. For example, your baby may be surprised or amused by your making up new silly verses to favorite songs, such as singing "The cows on the bus say moo, moo, moo" and then stopping and saying, "Wait a second! Cows on a bus? I don't think so! That's silly!"

Many babies also think the idea of things being "yucky" is quite amusing. You might try tasting each one of your baby's fingers and toes and finding some delicious ("like strawberries!") and others yucky ("like Brussels sprouts!"). Other things that are "wrong," such as trying hard to fit your baby's shoe on your foot or to wear it as your new hat, may be met with lots of giggles.

Looking to You for Information and Emotion Sharing

Your baby is starting to realize that you are her guide to the world, so watch her to see if she looks at you to judge your reaction to a new person or a new toy. At this age, she should also be starting to lift things up to show you so that you'll share in her excitement. If she doesn't do these things, get in the habit of moving your face into her sightline and showing her how you feel about these things (excited, happy, surprised, nervous, etc.).

Tool Use

Between 6 and 15 months babies get better at using "tools." From using a toy hammer to pound pegs to using a Velcro fishing rod to catch fuzzy fish to using a spoon to get food into their mouths, this is an important developmental milestone to encourage during these months.

Beginnings of Pretend Play

Babies are *just* beginning to understand the concept of pretend play. This is a good age at which to get your baby toy versions of things he sees you using, such as a vacuum cleaner or a lawn mower or a telephone. Pretend play is a way that children can start learning and rehearsing adult behaviors. However, another important function of pretend play is to help children emotionally process and put words to the things that happen to them. So a great way to introduce pretend play is to perform "instant replays" of things that just happened or that got a big emotional reaction from the baby. If your baby cried when Grandma jumped out and yelled "boo," put words to it ("You were scared!" or "Scary!") and then immediately have Teddy Bear cry when you jump out and yell "boo" ("Scary!"). If he loved being tossed up in the air—"Wheee!"—then toss up Teddy as he watches ("Wheee!!!") and pretend to have Teddy ask for "more" tossing.

Another great way to encourage pretend play is to "pretend" things with a doll while, or just after, your child does them. For example, you could set a place at the table for your child's doll or stuffed animal and pretend to feed the doll while your child is eating. After you give the doll a spoonful of imaginary food from her plate, hand the toy spoon to your child and see if she would like to have a turn feeding the baby. Pretending to feed the doll, change her diaper, and put her to sleep are good things to try, because these are all things with which your child has a lot of experience and is now very familiar. In the same way, driving and cooking are grown-up behaviors that your child has likely seen you do many times. For this reason, driving a pretend car using a laundry basket and a Frisbee steering wheel, or pretending to cook using a toy pot and spoon, or a small saucepan and wooden spoon from your kitchen, would be great things to pretend with your child.

Separation Anxiety

Younger babies have an easier time separating from their parents because for them it's "out of sight, out of mind," whereas older babies may begin to have difficulty with separation from caregivers. This is perfectly normal, and we offer a few tips for dealing with this.

First, never sneak out on your baby. Always say "Good-bye" and reassure her that you'll be back, or she may begin to wonder if you're going to leave unexpectedly. That can make babies anxious. Second, give her time to get comfortable in a new situation, at a new place, or with a new person, with you there. She'll see from your cues that you like this person or place, and she'll feel more comfortable. Third, give her a transition item of some kind, something that represents you and means you're coming back. This may be a special blankie, a stuffed animal, a pillow with your picture on it, or if separation at bedtime becomes difficult, something that smells like you, such as the shirt you've been wearing.

THINGS TO WATCH FOR

Each child develops at her own pace, but talk to your baby's doctor if your 12-month-old:

- seems to lose any skills or words she had previously mastered,
- does not frequently smile and often seems to have a "flat" facial expression,

- seems to lack interest in people; doesn't look you in the eye,
- does not use any gestures, like pointing or shaking her head no,
- avoids close contact or cuddling,
- becomes inconsolable for periods of longer than 30 minutes, or
- does not try to imitate any of your movements or sounds.

HOW YOU CAN HELP
YOUR 9- TO 12-MONTH-OLD LEARN

Here are some general principles:

- Continue the routines from previous sections that are still engaging to your baby.
- Play games in front of the mirror to encourage self-awareness.
- Give your child experience with other people and with animals so he can begin to grasp the idea that some things are living and some are not. You also want him to start getting the idea the living things have feelings, saying things like, "Doggie likes it when you pat him gently," or "Doggie really likes you. He wants you to pat him."
- Set up opportunities to point to things that will be really interesting to your child, like trips to see animals on a farm, aquarium, or zoo and trips to the playground to see other children.
- Make a set of personalized books for your child, as we described in Part II (for example, *What Does Baby Wear?* and *What Does Baby Eat?*).
- Although children may be a bit young for this, you can start to teach your child that things go in categories—for example, you could label "grapes," "cheese," "Cheerios," and say, "They're all yummy," or "They're all things to eat."
- This is a great time to start teaching your baby that he can make choices, so hold out two options for him, like a grape and a cracker, or a red sock and a blue sock, saying, "Which one?" or "Which one do you want?" and offer whichever one he reaches for.
- Now is the time to start singing some of his favorite songs and pausing before a last word, pausing during scripts of favorite games (for example, "Ready, set . . ."), and pausing during beloved books, waiting for the baby to "fill in the blank." You can also now begin to use pictures to represent real-world objects and allow your baby extra choices by making picture "menus" for everything from food to lullabies (see the facing page).
- Reinforce his attempts at communication (eye contact, word approximations, babbling at you, smiling, pointing at what he wants or wants to show you) by paying him lots of attention, looking happy, and giving him what he's requesting whenever possible.

Following are some specific activities you can do during daily routines.

Waking Up/Bedtime Routines

 UP?

When you see your baby in the morning, before you pick her up, say, "Up?" with your palms up and wait for the baby to reach for you. You're teaching her that words and gestures can mean the same thing. Then reinforce any attempt to communicate, like reaching her arms up, but if possible, require her to look at you while or just before you pick her up. If necessary, make it easy for her to look at you by squatting or standing in front of her just before you pick her up.

 WAKE UP, EVERYONE!

"Wake up" your baby's stuffed animals by greeting them good morning and saying, "Time to get out of bed!" As you and the baby make each one "jump" out of the crib, say, "Wake up, Elmo! Wake up, Teddy!" and so on. Go around the house helping your baby turn the lights on, saying, "Wake up, living room! Wake up, kitchen!" Give him as much help as needed to turn on the light switch and then reinforce this with praise ("You did it! You turned the light on!"), even if he needed help.

 NIGHT-NIGHT LULLABIES

Make one picture (cardboard works best, but you can use paper covered with plastic or laminated) to represent each of your baby's three favorite lullabies. At first, show her, for example, the "star" while you sing "Twinkle, Twinkle Little Star," the "sun" while you sing "You Are My Sunshine," and the "cradle" as you sing "Rock a Bye Baby" (see the drawings below). Then begin to show her two pictures at once to let her choose. Hold up the star and the sun pictures and say, "Do you want 'Twinkle, Twinkle' [as you shake the star] or 'You Are My Sunshine' [as you shake the sun]?" If she reaches for one, say, "Okay, 'Twinkle, Twinkle Little Star'!" and hand it to her and begin to sing it. If she doesn't make a choice, then you should choose one, hand it to her, and sing the song represented in the picture she is holding. Once she understands, she'll be able to choose her own lullaby. Once she has learned this, let her choose from all three pictures.

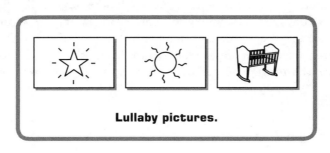

Lullaby pictures.

NIGHT-NIGHT, TEDDY!

Begin to tuck in all of your baby's stuffed animals at bedtime. Say, "Night-night, Teddy!" as you both kiss him and put him in or next to the crib and cover him with a blanket. This will help him understand the idea of pretend and get the idea that you're pretending Teddy is a real animal or child. If he can give Teddy a kiss or try to cover Teddy with a blankie (which can be a tissue, a washcloth, or a cloth diaper), give lots of praise ("What a good mommy [or daddy]! You put Teddy to bed!").

 BEDTIME READING

Hold up two books, one in each hand, and let your baby reach for the one she wants. At this age your baby may have memorized a few of her books and may have a few words or sounds that are close to words, although many children don't have any words until past their first birthday. Now you can begin to pause during your reading and wait for her to "fill in the blank." For example, "Now it's time to pat the . . . ," and then point to the bunny. If she makes any sound, she's probably trying to say "bunny," so go ahead and praise her: "Bunny! That's right! Hi, bunny!" You can also begin to ask her simple questions around her first words, like, "Who is that?" and wait for her to respond ("That's right, it's bunny!").

This is the age when children will lock on to a few books that they will likely want you to read over and over again until you are really bored with them. Although it can be tiresome for you, this is terrific practice for your baby's memory development.

 BABY'S OWN BOOKS

Make your own set of simple personalized books for your baby. For example, get a few small simple plastic photo albums from the dollar store and fill them with pictures of things in your baby's life. You can make a "Who Loves Baby?" book with one picture per page of important people in your lives. You can make a "What Does Baby Eat?" book with one picture per page of her favorite foods. You can make a "Where Does Baby Go?" book with one picture per page of important places you regularly go (playground, grocery store, etc.).

You can even make a whole book about a familiar routine. For example, if you bake cookies, you can take a picture at each stage and make one step per page, so that your baby can relive and rehearse the steps ("First we roll out the dough, then we . . ."). You could also try this with a routine you're having difficulty with, such as dropping off at day care or saying good night and leaving the room, so that your baby has a chance to process the emotions and the steps of this difficult routine in the safety of your arms. You could rehearse these steps during a relaxed time and also right before the routine actually happens, so your baby will be reminded of what to expect.

There are also recordable photo albums now, which allow you to record a short message on each page of the photo album. Having friends and relatives, such as grandparents, all record a short message with their pictures that the baby can press to hear their voices makes a wonderful teaching toy.

Create a memory book by taking one photo of your child each time you do something new or special such as having a playdate or going to a new playground. Then look back at the picture and talk about the experience in the days and weeks to come.

Feeding Time

 DRINKS FOR EVERYONE

When you get your baby's bottle, you could say, "A drink of milk for baby," and then get your coffee and say, "A drink of coffee for Mommy," and then go around watering the plants, saying, "A drink of water for this plant . . ."

 I MAKE MOMMY/DADDY HONK!

This is a silly contingency game (your behavior depends on your child's behavior) for when you are face to face at the table/high chair. Help your baby push your nose gently with his finger. As soon as he does, stick your tongue out. Hopefully he will giggle and keep pressing the "button" that makes your tongue stick out. When he begins to get bored, change it up. Start to make a "honk" sound every time he pushes your nose. When he gets bored, change the game again and give him a tickle each time he presses it. The variations on this game are endless. The point is to help him understand that his behavior brings about predictable consequences.

 FUN WITH FOOD! SQUISH, SQUISH!

Let your baby play with different-textured foods with her hands. For example, she might enjoy squishing Jell-O cubes through her fingers or painting with pudding or yogurt.

 WHERE IS IT HIDING?

When you have a small cracker, hide it in one of your hands in front of your baby, then put your hands behind your back and bring them out in front with your fists closed. If the baby touches one hand or reaches for it, open it. If it's empty, he'll go for the other hand. If it's full, he'll get the cracker. If he likes this game, try a simple pattern such as hiding in your left hand and then your right and then your left again, and see if he begins to catch on that you're going back and forth (problem solving!).

BABY'S FIRST WORDS

If there are a few words you're working on, tape a picture of each to the high chair tray or up next to the changing table. Then during these routines take an extra couple of opportunities to label and make a sign for the words while pointing to the picture by touching it. (For example, touch the picture of the flower, say "flower," and sniff.) This activity not only helps boost language development but also helps teach your baby the significance of pointing to something.

You can take out a knife and say "cut" each time you cut a piece of food in front of her, and you can make the pieces different sizes so that you can hold up two pieces and say, "Big piece or little piece? Oh, you want the big piece—here you go!" You can offer a few pieces of food at a time and count them when you put them down, for example, "Here's two—one, two." See Chapter 17 for other good words to start with.

 LET'S PRETEND!

Using a banana or a cup, begin to play "telephone." Make a "ring-ring" sound and pick up the "phone" and say, "Hello? Oh, hi, Grandpa! Baby, it's for you" (handing him the "phone"). Then prompt him to say, "Hi, Grandpa!" (or just make babbling sounds like ba-ba-ba da-da-da). Talking on the telephone is often one of the first kinds of pretend that children learn.

 WHICH ONE DO WE WANT?

Your baby may now be able to learn to make choices. Make a baby "menu" with pictures of her four favorite breakfast foods and ask her which one she wants. If she does not point to any of them, gently take her finger and touch it to one of the pictures and then say "Cheerios," and immediately give her some Cheerios.

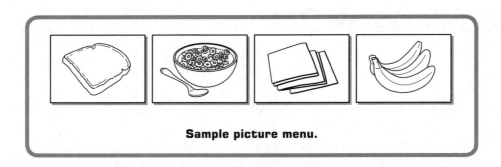

Sample picture menu.

I CAN FEED MYSELF!

Encourage fine motor development by serving small (non-choking-hazard) foods such as peas, baked beans, and the like. Show your baby how to pick up one at a time.

Diaper Changing and Dressing

 CAN I HAVE IT?

Bring your baby close to the diapers, point to them, and say, "Can you get a diaper?" Then you might put out your hand and look at him expectantly, saying, "Can Daddy have it?" Make this as easy as possible by just having a pile of two or three diapers, or even just one, within easy reach. If he doesn't respond, you could put a diaper in his hand and help him hand it to you, then give him a big thank you.

 WHICH SOCKS?

If you're changing her clothes, begin to hold up two sets of pants or socks and ask, "Which one do you want?" and when she reaches, say, "Oh, you want the blue ones!" If she doesn't reach out, you can gently take her hand and make it touch one option and *then* say, "Oh, you want the blue ones!" (With practice she'll learn that the choice she touches is the one she'll get.)

 SHIRT ON, SHIRT OFF

As you undress your baby, say things like, "The shirt is ON." Then pull it off: "The shirt is OFF! Oh, look, it's your little tummy! I love your little tummy!" (Give tummy kisses.) "The sock is ON . . . the sock is OFF! Oh, look, it's your little foot! I love your little foot!" (Give feet kisses.) If your baby is enjoying this, you can pause and wait for eye contact before you give the tickly kisses.

 WHERE'S BABY'S ARM?

Play hide and seek with your baby's body parts while getting him dressed. As you put his shirt over his head, say, "Where is Baby's head?" As you pull his head through, say, "Here it is!" Play this with arms and hands going through sleeves and legs and feet going through pants.

 DIAPER SONG

Sing any song your child likes while you change her diaper. Stop any time your child's attention wanders. As soon as she makes eye contact with you, begin singing again. This is one of those games where your baby's eye contact makes the game, song, or action start or continue.

SILLY MOMMY/DADDY!

Always be looking for opportunities to be silly and share a laugh. At changing/ dressing time, this could mean trying to put the baby's tiny baby shoe on your big foot or pretending you have mistaken it for your new hat.

Bathtime

 MOMMY/DADDY SAYS

This game is almost like "Simon Says"—however, in the baby version, you never try to trick the baby by leaving out the Simon Says part. Take a few actions that your baby already knows how to do (for example, clap hands, pat head, bang a cup on the tub), and say, "Mommy says touch your head," while patting your own head. As soon as the baby pats his head, say, "Yay! Mommy says bang the cup" as you bang the cup. If he doesn't try to imitate you, gently take his hand and make it do the action, then enthusiastically praise him ("You did it! Yay!") and perhaps give him a little splash or tickle if he likes that.

 SPLASH WITH YOUR FEET

Try teaching your baby to "splash" with different body parts. Take her feet and gently kick them in the water, saying, "Splash with your feet," and then take her hands and say, "Splash with your hands." Next, you can take a bath crayon and draw some little people or animals on the side of the tub and show them how to "splash doggie," "splash bunny," and so on. When you erase them, say, "Good-bye, doggie, good-bye bunny." After you've demonstrated, give the instruction again, like, "Good-bye, doggie," and then give as much help as needed for the child to erase the doggie, like pointing to the doggie or directing your child's hand toward it. When she erases it, no matter how much help she needed, praise her enthusiastically.

If you have some small tub animals, line them up on the side of the bath and have each one jump into the bath, saying, "Jump, splash!" and then do it again, adding the animal names: "Froggy, jump, splash; duck, jump, splash," and so on.

 READY, SET, GO!

If you have any wind-up toys for the bath, use them to teach the phrase "Ready, set, go!" pulling the string to make the duck or boat go on the "go," and then use simple phrases to describe what's happening: "The duck is swimming, the boat is sailing." If your child is starting to make some wordlike sounds or even words, you can do this a few times, then wind up a toy, say, "Ready, set . . . ," and wait for the child to try to say "go" or "g," then let the wind-up toy go.

IN AND OUT

If you have a baby basketball net, or a net for cleaning up bath toys, try putting different bath toys in the net with the word "in" (then the second time you do it, name the objects—"ball in, cup in," etc.). If something is too big, say, "Oops—too big!" Then ask your baby if you should take them all out ("Froggy out? Okay, Froggy out"). Cups that nest inside one another are also terrific for teaching "in" and "out" as you help your baby put them all inside one another and then take them all out again.

 DRY AND WET

When you first put your baby in the bath, most of his body will be dry. Again, use simple, repetitive phrases to teach these concepts: "Now baby's tummy is dry . . . [then, pouring some water onto his tummy] now it's wet!" You can use the same phrasing to demonstrate wet and dry with your washcloths and sponges (sponges are great because they can be wet and then instantly dry again).

 STICKS/DOESN'T STICK

There are lots of foam letters/vehicles/animals that are meant to stick to the side of the tub. You can try teaching your baby to put these up on the wall, saying, "It sticks!" and also mix in some regular bath toys that won't stick. When you put those up, say, "Doesn't stick," or "Oops—it fell down" (and laugh when the toys hit the water—anything you laugh at will hold more interest for your baby). Get her involved by handing her things to try sticking on the side of the tub, prompting with as much help as she needs.

 BODY PARTS

Using bubble bath or bath foam (consistency of shaving cream), place bubbles or cream on different parts of your body and your baby's body, labeling "Mommy's nose, Baby's nose," and offering choices: "Should I put it on your hand or your belly?" Point and then wipe it off and say, "All gone." Wait for the baby to indicate some body part by touching or pointing to it; if he doesn't, help him touch one body part, like his belly. As you soap each part of baby's body, sing about it to a familiar tune (for example, to "The Wheels on the Bus," sing "Now I'm washing Baby's feet, Baby's feet, Baby's feet"), then repeat the verses for rinsing, drying, and rubbing lotion onto each body part. You can end by offering tickles and kisses for each body part.

 PRETEND

Do the same thing as above, but on a waterproof animal or character toy, so that your baby sees Elmo getting the same scrub-down and gets a chance to hear all the same words again. Again, ask her which body part to wash ("Elmo's foot or Elmo's tummy?") and put the washcloth wherever she points or touches. If she doesn't choose a body part, help her choose one by putting her hand or finger on Elmo and saying, "Oh, you want the tummy! Okay, let's wash Elmo's tummy." If she keeps choosing the same body part, that's okay; keep washing what she chooses.

 SINK AND FLOAT

Get a bucket of various objects and let the baby drop them in the tub, observing whether they "sink" or "float." Another way to play is to make floating boats out of aluminum foil ("float") and then see how many figurines, bathtub letters or numbers, or other toys it takes to sink them ("sink").

 COLORS

A drop of food coloring or some fizzy colored bath tablets can be really fun in the bath. Take any opportunity you can to let the baby make a choice, so hold up two different colors and when he reaches for one say, "Oh, you want the red one." Drop in the tablet or food coloring and give him a big wooden spoon to stir the color in (repetitive songs tend to get babies' attention—songs like "Mix-a mix-a mix-a till our bath-a bath-a bath-a turns all red-a red-a red-a"). Then praise him—"Wow, you did it! You turned your bath red!"—and find more ways to reinforce the concept of red such as sorting red and non-red things: "I'm going to get all of our red bath toys. Here's a red one; it goes in the bath. Oops, not red [leave it out]. Red. Not red." Then when you get out of the bath, see if you can keep it going by finding, for example, a red blanket, a red towel, or red pajamas. Your baby is too young to learn words for colors, but you're giving him a head start by calling his attention to colors that are similar and another opportunity to make a choice.

Doing Errands/Going for a Walk

 HELP MOMMY/DADDY SHOP

While you're grocery shopping, hand your baby groceries to put in the cart as you say "Put in." As you do this, you can name them or talk about them: "Apples—you love apples!" "These cans are heavy!" Then reinforce his attempt to help you (even if you needed to help him put it in the cart with your hand over his hand): "What a good helper! Thank you!"

 WHICH ONE DO YOU WANT?

Hold up two choices for the baby—for example, two different kinds of cereals or apples—and say, "Which one do you want?" and let her put the one she wants in the cart. This is excellent practice in making and communicating a choice. After she's mastered this, if she's close to a year old, you can encourage her to start pointing to the one she wants or touching it with her index finger, instead of just reaching for it. If the food is something that you can open and give her a small piece of (like one Cheerio), even better! That's a great reinforcer for having made a choice!

 WORD OF THE DAY

Each time you take a walk with a stroller, think about one word or concept on which to focus. Will you push the stroller "fast" and "slow"? Will you point out everything red? Will you point out every mailbox? Every set of Christmas lights? Every dog? (Note that this can work in other contexts too, such as finding lots of things to "squeeze" one day or to "push" the next day. Also, see "theme days" in Chapter 3.)

Chores Around the House

 LAUNDRY TIME AND HELPING MOMMY COOK

"Laundry Time" and "Helping Mommy Cook" (see Chapter 15) may be even more fun for your baby at this age. You can try a variety of sizes and shapes of wooden spoons and small pots. You could also give your baby a few small bits of choke-proof food that he likes (for example, a few Cheerios) and encourage him to drop them in the pot and stir them around.

 WASH THE CAR

If you're doing yard work or washing your car, give your baby a watering can to help you water the plants or a bucket of water and some waterproof dolls or animal figures and let her give them a "bath." Or give her a small bucket of water and a sponge and a toy car, and she can wash the toy car while you wash the real one. And, of course, she can help you wash the real one too. Show her how to scrub with the sponge, back and forth or in a circular motion. Praise her for any attempt to help you wash the car or her toy.

 PAINT THE HOUSE

Another fun thing to keep your baby entertained while you do yard work is to give her a paintbrush and a bucket of water and let her "paint" the house, deck, or driveway with water. This will help keep her busy as well as strengthening the idea of imitating adults. Give her lots of praise for helping and an occasional kiss or cuddle. Or you can give her a little plastic toy rake and have her work alongside you, raking, picking up sticks and putting them in a big bucket, and imitating any of your movements and activities that she can.

WHAT DO I HEAR?

As you turn on anything with a sound, such as your water faucet, blender, vacuum cleaner, or coffee maker, you can cup your hand to your ear and say, "I hear a _____!" You can place noisy toys on the baby's high chair or in the baby's play area so that you can continue to label: "I hear a piano! I hear a squeaky rubber duck!" You can also make different sounds as you clean, such as a sneeze, a cough, a yawn, labeling each time "I heard a _____!" Alternatively, you can record a series of familiar sounds and then play the recording while you cook dinner or shower, stating after each sound, "I hear a cow! I hear a cat! I hear bath water! I hear the car! I hear the telephone!"

Playtime

 LET'S DRAW!

Babies will start to be interested in watching you draw as you narrate (for example, "Circle, circle, circle, eyes, nose, mouth . . . look, it's a snowman!" whether this is with crayons, with markers on a mirror, on a chalkboard, etc.). They will also be ready to begin trying to make their own scribbles on paper with crayons.

Place some finger paints in zipper bags and lay them flat in front of your baby in his high chair or on the floor and show him how to draw in the paint with his fingers and squish the paint around inside the bags. Alternatively, put some paper on the bottom of a rectangular plastic food storage container, squirt on some paint, and toss in a couple of marbles, and then seal the container with the lid and let the baby "paint" by shaking and rolling the marbles around the container. The interesting visual effects will be a natural reinforcer for participating in this activity.

 LET'S TALK!

Once your child starts to babble, you can encourage him to imitate your babbling by doing it into a coffee can or paper towel holder or something that creates an interesting echo. You can also take turns making silly sounds into a child's tape recorder and then move on to words. This is a really enticing way to begin teaching her to imitate your sounds and words. You say something into the toy and play it back and then give her a turn. You want her to make successively better imitations of your sounds and words. If your child has favorite people, toys, foods, or books, she might think it's fun to start practicing saying the words for those favorite things. Praise any attempt to imitate your words.

 BABY BASKETBALL

Start with a large basket like a laundry basket right in front of your baby and a bucket or box full of balls. You can also show your baby how to make his own balls by crumpling up paper (which is fun on its own). Show the baby how you throw balls into the laundry basket, saying, "He shoots! He scores!" or "Oops!" Hold out your hand palm up and ask him to get the balls for you. He can retrieve and give them to you, with your help if needed. You can build anticipation by saying, "Ready, set, go!" and moving the basket "near" and "far." If he is starting to say words, you can pause after "Ready, set," and wait for him to try to say "go." If the baby is interested, help him "throw" the balls into the basket right in front of him. As he gets older, you can keep this game challenging by moving the basket farther away.

 BALLOONS

Be very careful never to let a small child near balloons unsupervised, because of the choking hazard. You can blow up a balloon, say, "Ready, set, go!" and let it fly around the room. If your baby finds that funny and exciting, do it a few more times, then pause after "Ready, set . . . ," and wait for her to make an attempt to say "go" or just make some noise and look at you, then say, "Go!" and let it fly! If she goes to pick it up, let her hand it to you as a way to request doing it again, but make sure you're right there so she doesn't put it in her mouth. Some children find this game a bit scary. In that case, you could blow it up less full so it doesn't fly as fast or as far and do it at a greater distance from the baby. If she's still scared, or cries, just move on to something else. With helium balloons, try putting a couple in a box and letting the baby shut the box and then open it, releasing the balloons so they float to the ceiling. Then pack them back up and do it again. Use simple language to describe what's happening: "Look! The balloons are going up, up, up! Now let's pull them down, down, . . . !" Pause to see if your baby will fill in by saying "da"; since most babies have no words at this age, if she doesn't attempt to say the first sound of the word, just fill it in for her.

 WHERE'S YOUR NOSE?

At first you can ask the baby, "Where's your nose?" and then kiss it and say, "Here it is. Kiss nose." You can do this for other body parts, like ears, cheeks, chin, hair, forehead, arms, hands, ending with "Where's your tummy?" and then tickling it, saying, "Here it is!" As your baby gets used to this game you can help him point to his body parts in response to your question. Then you can switch it up, saying, "Where's MY nose?" helping the baby point to your nose or give it a kiss by putting it up to his lips. If he doesn't reply accurately yet, just prompt him to touch the correct body part and then reinforce with a kiss just as you would if he had needed no help. The reward or reinforcer is the tummy tickle at the end when you ask, "Where's your . . . TUMMY?" and the fun comes from the fact that your child never knows when you will ask that particular question.

 NOTHING CAN GO WRONGO

"Nothing can go wrongo. I am in the Congo." Raffi has a song with this lyric, but feel free to make up any rhyme you like. Try drumming slowly on anything that makes noise, even the floor, while slowly saying this line, and then make the beat faster and faster as you say it faster and faster. Next follow the baby's rhythm. When she drums slowly, say the line slowly, and when she drums fast, say the line fast. She'll enjoy controlling your tempo.

 LET'S UNWRAP

If you have extra wrapping paper around, try wrapping some of your baby's toys loosely and letting him have the fun of unwrapping them or ripping off the paper. Say things like, "Hmm. What could it be? Oh, it's a _____!" Tissue paper works especially well for this because it tears very easily. When your baby receives gifts for his birthday or for another special occasion, he will have had some practice at opening his own presents.

 WHERE'S MOMMY/DADDY?

This is an auditory tracking game. Once your baby can move around a bit, by crawling or scooting on her behind, try hiding yourself (behind a chair, wall, or curtain, under a blanket, etc.) as you continuously say, "Where is Mommy?" and letting her find you by tracking your voice. **Of course, be sure to keep an eye on what she's doing and where she's going!**

 STICKS, DOESN'T STICK

Get some sticky contact paper and stick some of your baby's toys to it. Then place some of his other toys on the floor next to it. When he pulls on the toys stuck to the contact paper, say, "Sticks!" When he picks up a toy from the floor, say, "Doesn't stick!" You can put other easy language to this game, like "That's hard!" and "That's easy!" Find a magnetic surface (for example, the fridge or dishwasher) and gather some magnetic and nonmagnetic objects. Take turns picking up an object and saying either "Sticks!" or "Doesn't stick" when it's nonmagnetic and falls down.

 SAND TABLE OR SANDBOX

You can hide toy figures in the sand and say, "Where did _____ go?" You can pretend to look everywhere and then finally help your baby dig the figure out of the sand, saying, "Oh! There it is!" This will help him build his concept of object permanence (things still exist when they go out of sight). Finding the toys hidden in the sand is a great natural reinforcer for the activity of looking, so be sure to give your baby a few minutes to enjoy playing with them. And you can do the same thing indoors with a large bin of rice, lentils, or beans. Playing in sand and water at the beach is a really special treat. Help your baby make a cake, and then you can place sticks in the sand-cake and pretend they are candles and sing "Happy Birthday" and "blow out the candles." Note that at this age it is good to begin asking your baby more questions, even if you're the one who has to answer them. Pretend you're baking sand-cookies and ask, "What kind of cookies are you making? Chocolate chip? Mmmm!"

 STACKING RINGS, BLOCKS, PUZZLES

Name the colors as you stack them together and practice the words "on" and "off." Put on ring bracelets and ring hats to be silly. Teach your baby to "build them up . . . and knock them down!" by letting the baby take turns with you building and knocking down towers of rings or blocks. This is also a good time to introduce two- to three-piece form board puzzles to do together. Try simple language like "Fits!" or "Oops! Doesn't fit!"

 TUG OF WAR

Get something like a small blanket, roll it up, and have baby pull on one side while you pull on the other. Pretend to pull back and forth for a minute before pretending to fall over: "Boom!" This should get lots of giggles. Giggling time is also a great time to get good eye contact by placing yourself in front of baby while she's laughing.

 LET'S SWING

Swinging is an easy activity for teaching extended eye contact. Push your baby from the front on a baby swing where he is well supported and then stop the swing and wait for him to look at you before pushing again.

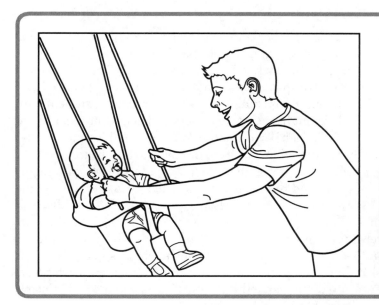

If your child breaks off eye contact while swinging, hold the swing near you until he looks at you again and then resume pushing.

GENERAL FACTORS THAT PROMOTE HEALTHY BRAIN DEVELOPMENT

In addition to playing and teaching, there are a few factors under your control that can help optimize your baby's brain development. First, exercise and sunshine are not only helpful for babies' sleep cycles, but encourage the production of a chemical called "brain-derived neurotropic factor," which helps to support the survival of existing neurons and encourage the growth and differentiation of new neurons and synapses. In addition, adequate protein intake and a variety of vitamins and minerals from iron to vitamin D can affect everything from cognitive development to mood. After he starts on solid food, be sure to give your baby foods with protein, like milk, yogurt, or small portions of meat, and fruits or vegetables (preferably both) for vitamins. If you have questions about complete nutrition, protecting against sunburn, or possible allergies, ask your pediatrician.

Other games you can play while he's swinging are pretending that he's knocking you down by letting his feet just touch you as he swings toward you and then falling back in an exaggerated way, saying, "Bonk!" Or you can duck out of the way as he comes toward you, pretending each time that it's a "Close one—whew!"

Play peekaboo while you push the baby in a baby swing. Push him gently away and then cover your face with your hands or a cloth and then uncover your face when he swings back toward you, saying, "Here I am!" This should be funny to him and help him focus on your face.

 TREASURE HUNT

Go on hunts for lots of examples of the same thing or same characteristic. For example, find and collect all the balls in your child's play area, or all the books, or all the cups, or all the toy ducks. Label each of them. This will help your child form categories—in other words, to learn that cups are not simply objects that are blue, like his favorite sippy cup, but that everything with a similar shape can be a cup. You can even try having two different boxes or containers and help your child figure out which should go where ("Is this a ball or a book? Where should we put it?").

You can also take different-colored mats, cloth, or construction paper and help your baby hunt for things around the house that "match." For example, you might put down a yellow piece of paper and then search the kitchen for something yellow ("Hmm. What is yellow? Is an apple yellow? No. Is a spoon yellow? No. Is a banana yellow? YES!"), then bring a banana back and put it on the paper and say, "Yellow! Match!" and then search the bathroom for something yellow and find a rubber duckie to bring back, and so on. Give your baby as much help as she needs to put the object in the right place and then praise her for great matching, no matter how much help was needed. You can do the same thing with a Twister game mat, placing a different object on each circle of the matching color.

PART IV

MORE TIPS AND TOOLS

CHAPTER 17

Specific Words, Phrases, Gestures, and Signs to Work On

In this chapter we're going to suggest some categories of words and phrases that many children learn early in the process of acquiring language, as well as some examples within each category. We will also touch on simple gestures and signs that the child can make with his hands (more baby signs can be found online). If there are words or phrases that are frequently used in your family that are not on the list in this chapter, just add those, and if there are words or phrases that your child would not hear very often, just forget about those. These are all just suggestions.

Children use single words first and usually begin with words they hear often or the names of people and objects that are important to them. Using those words frequently will encourage your child to learn them. Using the same single words often, pointing to or showing the objects they label, and responding immediately when your child attempts to use a word he has heard (even if it does not sound quite like the word) are all good ways to use these lists.

Once children have mastered a few single words, they will begin to combine them into simple phrases to communicate something they want or do not want. That's why the first phrases are often "more _____" or "no _____." (The signs for both are shown later in this chapter. Also see the box on page 192 for a note about "more.")

The strategies discussed throughout the book will be helpful in teaching these words and simple phrases. Use the word you want to teach often so that your child begins to understand what it refers to; use the filling-in method and wait for your child to use the word. Most important, respond immediately when your child attempts to communicate. You're teaching him to use language as a tool at the same time that you're teaching him new words and phrases.

191

USING THE "MORE" SIGN

Here's one thing to keep in mind if you teach your child to make the sign for "more": Although most early interventionists do teach this sign, some children just learn to make this sign whenever they want something. The problem with this is that the adults may not be able to figure out what the child wants, which can be very frustrating for everyone. In addition, it may discourage the child from learning more effective ways to communicate what he wants, such as pointing to the object or saying the first sound of the word. So if you teach the sign for "more," try to use it only when your child wants you to continue a fun activity or wants more of a good thing you're giving him. And definitely encourage him to make his requests specific, by pointing to what he wants, saying the word or the first sound of the word, or making the sign for the word, like "eat" (depicted on page 201).

UNDERSTANDING VERSUS SAYING

When you're teaching your child to say words, the general idea is to model the word for the child by saying it clearly and with lots of emphasis, like "baNAna," while showing the child a banana or a picture of a banana. If she can imitate you, you should very enthusiastically praise her using simple words, like "Great talking. It's a baNAna." Beginning by teaching your child the names of the things she likes most should increase her motivation to try to say them. Teaching children to use words to request the things they want, and then responding by immediately giving them the things they've requested, is a terrific way to show them what a powerful tool speech can be. And remember to reinforce any effort your child makes to say the word. If she can say only a very rough approximation of the word, like "nana" or even "na" for "banana" or "bubba" or "ba" for "bubbles," that's fine—it's the effort and the approximation that you want to reward. The more your child is willing and eager to try to say words, the more practice she will get with her articulation and the better it will become.

It's more difficult to judge whether a child really *understands* a word or phrase than whether he can say it. This is because you can hear him say the word or an approximation of the word, and it's pretty clear that he does or does not have a consistent sound for the object (like "nana" for "banana" or "bubba" for "bubbles"). However, when he seems to understand the word when you say it, he may be using the situation or context to understand what you're saying instead of the actual word. For example, if you say, "Do you want a banana?" while you're holding up the banana, he may understand that you're offering the banana and reach for it, or push it away if he doesn't want it, without really understanding the *word* "banana."

In the daily routines in Part II that list language as a target skill, we give you a lot of examples of activities you can use to teach your child to understand simple words and phrases. (You can use the Index or the Appendix to identify the ones that specifically target language.) In this chapter we just list the simple words and phrases you might wish to introduce as you move through your day so your child can eventually understand and produce them. As with everything else you want to teach, don't tackle too much at once. It's best to pick a few words from each category and give your child lots of opportunities to hear and, if possible, produce those words.

WORDS

Animals

Many children learn animal names or sometimes the noise the animal makes at an early age. Some of the most common are:

cat (or kitty) (meow)	cow (moo)
dog (or doggy) (woof)	pig (oink)
bird	fish
horse (neigh)	duck (quack)
sheep (baa)	chicken

Vehicles

Use the names or the sounds of vehicles that your child is likely to ride in, or see frequently, or for which she has a toy version (like a toy truck).

car (vroom vroom)	airplane
truck	bus
train (choo choo)	boat

Toys

Use the ones your child is familiar with or add your own. Favorite toys are particularly good to use.

ball	teddy bear
puzzle	doll
book	

Body Parts

tummy (or belly or whatever word you use)	head
eyes	hair
nose	arm
mouth	foot
ear	knee
hand	leg

Clothing

jacket	hat
shirt	gloves (or mittens)
pants	sweater
dress	pajamas
socks	diaper
shoes	

Feelings

happy	scared
sad	silly/funny
mad (or angry)	

Outdoors

swing	car (or bus or train if he rides in one more often)
slide	go outside
playground	park
go home	store

People

Use whatever word you have for these people.

Mommy	Grandma
Daddy	Grandpa
Name of child's sister or brother	Name of friend or neighbor (child or adult) the child sees often
Name of other relatives (for example, Aunt Sue, cousin Sam)	Name of teacher if she has one

Food

This will vary a lot from family to family depending on what you eat. Use the words for foods and drinks that the child is most likely to see often. Try to use simple words. Here are some examples, but this really has to be picked by you to fit your life:

milk	fruit (blueberries, apple, peach, plum, etc.)
juice	
water	vegetables (carrots, peas, etc.)
Cheerios (or specific cereal the child likes and gets)	applesauce
	cracker
yogurt	cookie
cheese	chips
jelly	bread
rice	macaroni or spaghetti

Things around the House

spoon	blanket
bowl	crib
plate	bed
cup	pillow
bottle	phone
towel	chair
potty	table
tub	door
comb or brush	window
toothbrush	couch

Daily Activities

bath	bye (or bye-bye)
clean-up	nap (or naptime)
lunch, breakfast, dinner, supper, snack	peekaboo, hide and seek (or other favorite game)
night-night	change diaper
hi	get dressed

Describing and Other Words

big	off
little	uh-oh/oops
soft	yucky
hard	yummy
cold	wet
hot	dry
red, green, blue, etc.	down
fast	up
slow	yes
on	no

Action Words

run	wipe	feed
walk	stop	cook
sit	go	swing
stand up	open	wash
push	close	dry
hug	ride	read
kiss	eat	say
throw	drink	touch
catch	give	

PHRASES TO WORK ON

All done (can be alone or with
  another word, like "all done
  bath," "all done lunch")

More (preferably with another word,
  like "more Cheerios," "more
  bubbles")

____, please ("Cheerios, please,"
  "bubbles, please")

I want ____, please ("I want
  Cheerios, please"; "I want
  bubbles, please")

Go ____ (go car, go playground, go
  outside, go potty, go night-night)

Take out

Put in

Fall down

Person's ____ (Mommy's cup or
  Mommy cup, Baby's hat or Baby
  hat, Mommy's car or Mommy
  car, Sibling's book or Sibling
  book)

Where's Mommy? (where's book,
  where's apple). "Where" and
  "what" are usually the first
  questions that children learn to
  ask, and "where" is easier to
  teach.

GESTURES

points (see special section below on
  teaching pointing)

give me (hold out your hand and say
  "give me" and praise the child for
  putting the object in your hand)

waves bye-bye

pretends to feed a baby doll or
  stuffed animal

pretends to put a baby doll or
  stuffed animal to bed

raises arms to be picked up

pretends to stir a pot

pretends to talk on the phone (puts
  phone to ear and says a word or
  babbles)

pretends to drink from an empty cup

kisses a baby doll or stuffed animal

pretends to dress or diaper a baby
  doll or stuffed animal

pushes a toy car

SIGNS

The following are signs you can teach your child for useful requests the child will
want to make. Some of these can be found on line (*www.babysignlanguage.com*) as
part of baby signing, and some are modifications of American Sign Language (click
on "first 100 signs" at *www.lifeprint.com*). As we note in Chapter 18, having a way
to communicate these needs and desires when the child does not yet have language
can head off frustration and problem behavior. Chapter 18 offers ideas for reinforcing the use of whatever means of communication the child can manage and also
offers alternative ways to communicate besides using words or signs.

HELP

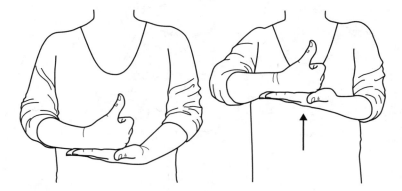

ALL DONE

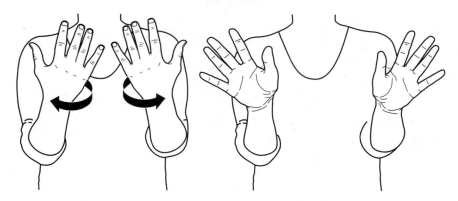

BREAK

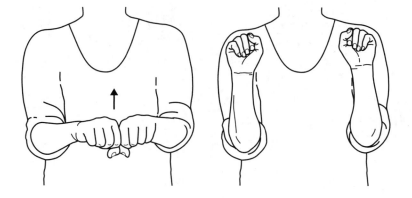

MORE

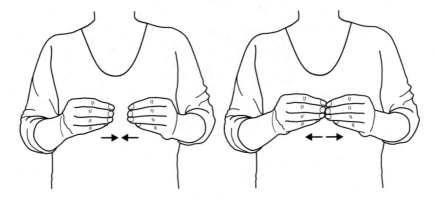

I WANT

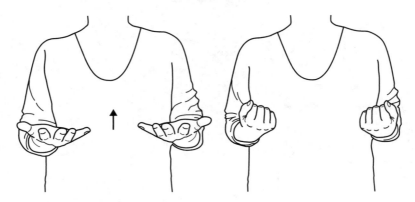

PUSH

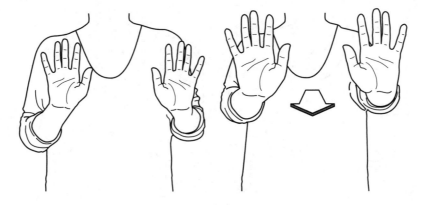

GO

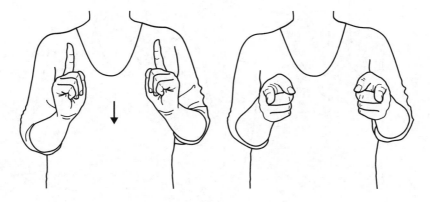

FLOWER

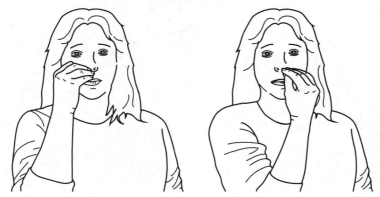

BABY

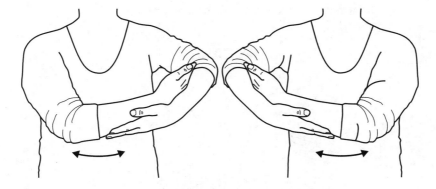

NO

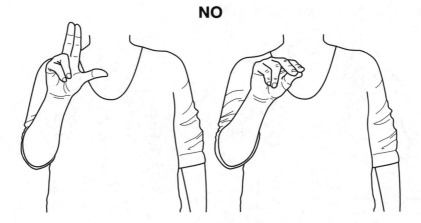

A simpler variation is described in Chapter 18. Your child can also simply shake his head.

YES

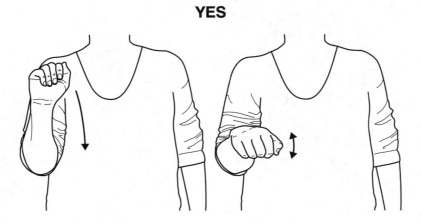

An alternative is to teach your child to just nod her head.

PLEASE

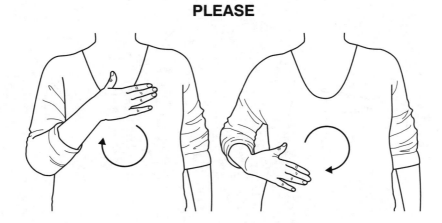

STOP

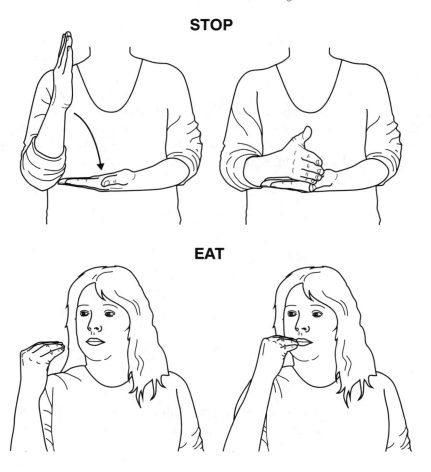

EAT

TEACHING YOUR CHILD TO POINT

We've referred to the importance of pointing often in this book, and now we want to review the basic steps for teaching pointing. If your child can point to what she wants, that will be a great first step in developing specific communication skills. When she cries and fusses, she may be communicating that she's unhappy, hungry, or uncomfortable—*but* if she can point to the cookie she wants or the dog that she fears, she is communicating a very specific need or desire. This will be an important step not only in developing communication, but also in preventing some problem behaviors that may arise when your child can't communicate what she wants and needs.

You can start with having a preferred food or a very attractive toy available but out of reach. For example, you could put the toy on a shelf where it can be seen or seat your child in a high chair and hold the toy or snack just out of his reach but in clear view. When the child reaches for the toy or treat, gently help him form a point with your other hand and have the child touch or almost touch the thing he wants (see the drawing below). Then immediately say something like, "Oh, you want the cookie [or the toy]. Here it is." Then give it to him. If it's an edible treat, make it a small piece so you can repeat this several times without his getting tired of the treat. If it's a toy, it's best to begin using a toy that has several pieces so that you don't need to take the toy away from him each time you want to give him another opportunity to practice pointing. Toys like puzzles, blocks, stacking rings or cups, shape sorters, Mr. Potato Head, or any other assembly toys your child enjoys will work well for this. Each time he points to the thing he wants, immediately reinforce that behavior by praising him and giving him what he requested by pointing.

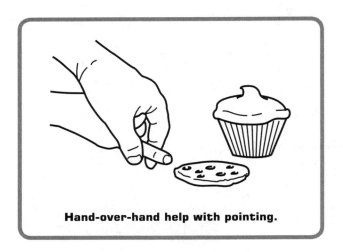

Hand-over-hand help with pointing.

As with other behavioral teaching, be sure to fade your physical prompts as soon as you can. For example, after you've physically prompted your child to point to what she wants a few times, try pausing for a couple of seconds to see if she will start to point by herself. Give her only as much help as she needs. If she starts to extend her pointer finger but doesn't fold in her other fingers to form a true point, praise her for the attempt while helping her complete the point. After she has started to extend her finger and touch the object she wants, you can help her point from a little distance instead of actually touching the object. Catch her when she's pointing to, but not yet touching, the object and then praise her: "Good pointing!" or "Oh, you want cookie!" as you hand her the treat.

Be patient! Although most children learn to point by around a year old, some children have a lot of difficulty getting the idea of pointing to what they want but can learn it slowly over time. Give your child lots of practice by doing this many times a day and make sure to practice using highly preferred treats or toys so that your child is very motivated to get them. ***But* be sure to switch it up or give him a rest at the first signs of frustration or boredom.**

You can also help your child understand how helpful pointing can be by pointing to things she likes or may find interesting throughout the day and directing her attention to those things. You can encourage her to follow your point to look at things you are looking at and then encourage her to point to show you things as well as to request them. Whenever your child shows you something, be sure to respond with enthusiasm, even if you had prompted her to do it in the first place. This will help your child begin to use communication not only to obtain objects that she wants but also to share her experience and enjoy and pay attention to what other people are doing.

CHAPTER 18

Preventing Problem Behavior

If your child has significant problem behaviors, like deliberately hurting himself, making real attempts to hurt other people or animals, making serious attempts to destroy other people's things (beyond the occasional 2-year-old tantrum), or having tantrums that go on for hours, it's best to get professional help to set up and manage a behavior program. Ask your child's doctor to recommend a local behavioral intervention program that can help you. And when it comes to problem behavior, the sooner you begin with a high-quality intervention program the better. However, some children have behavior problems that are less serious—occasional tantrums where a child may throw himself on the floor, scream, kick, thrash around, and cry or, even less serious than that, whining, throwing things to the ground, or simply refusing to do things when asked. If that is the case with your child, thinking about problem behavior as a means of communication and then helping your child find alternative means of communication may prove helpful. Furthermore, thinking about your child's behavior in this way can help to prevent serious problem behavior from developing in the first place; that is our main focus here.

All babies communicate to adults by fussing and crying (in addition to smiling and cooing). This is the only way they have to communicate that they need something. As they begin to learn to communicate in more mature and specific ways, like pointing, using other gestures (like lifting arms to be picked up), or using words, they cry and fuss less often.

But what about children who are having a harder time learning to communicate effectively about what they need and how they feel? Crying and fussing often remain the only forms of communication available to these children. They may feel very frustrated when they can't clearly communicate what they need. In addition, some children have a "slow to warm up" temperament and are overly sensitive to changes in their environment and may get very upset when offered a new, instead of a familiar, food or when they see a change in their routine or their home. See the box below for more on how to introduce new things.

EASING INTO CHANGE

If your child has difficulty with new things, it's important to try to help her acclimate to change. Here are a few ideas:

1. You can try introducing one new thing—such as a new song or a new book—sandwiched between two old favorites when she is a "captive audience" such as when she's in the bathtub or in the car seat on a trip.

2. You can attempt to pair change with something safe and beloved—for example, moving a piece of furniture in your living room and then immediately sitting and snuggling with the baby and his favorite lovey or snack in the new spot or keeping a special toy in the closet and bringing it out only when new people come to your home, or offering a large bite of a favorite food right after a tiny bite of a new food.

3. You can also allow your baby extra time to get used to new or overwhelming stimuli. For example, you might ask your pediatrician to first listen to your heartbeat and then listen to a teddy bear's heartbeat before placing the stethoscope on the baby's chest to listen to his heartbeat. Or you might find that if you leave a new toy in the middle of the living room for a few days, showing your child briefly once in a while how you play with it, she'll eventually approach it and try it.

Most children learn to cry less and communicate in other ways as they grow. Children who have difficulty learning language and communication may learn to cry more, and they may learn other kinds of behavior that help them communicate their displeasure or frustration with not being able to get the things they want and need. These behaviors might include screaming, hitting, kicking, or throwing things to the ground. When children do these things, their parents may rush to try to figure out what they need and give it to them. In this way, crying as a means of communication is followed by reinforcement, while other methods of communication are not being learned, practiced, or reinforced. If you think about what you've learned so far in this book about how reinforcement strengthens the behavior that it follows, it isn't difficult to understand how problem behavior can develop, even as early as 2 or 3 years of age.

TEACHING YOUR CHILD TO COMMUNICATE WHAT HE WANTS AND NEEDS

So what can you do in this situation? **The main solution is to figure out what the child is trying to communicate and teach him a better way to communicate it. Probably the single most important skill a child can learn, for the prevention of problem behavior, is how to communicate requests effectively.** So much problem behavior becomes unnecessary when parents understand what their children want and need. However, it is important to remember that some children find it hard to make requests nicely once they become upset, even if they know how. This is especially true if the skill of making requests is new and still requires considerable effort and attention. For this reason it's a very good idea to prompt your child to make a request at the very first sign that he's getting frustrated or upset, without waiting for him to get really upset.

You can do this in many ways:

- You can ask your child to show you what he wants (using pointing or gestures).
- If your child uses pictures to communicate, you can hand her the board with her picture choices and say, "Show me what you want." Or, if you think you know what she wants, you could hand her a picture of whatever it is you think she wants and say, "Is this what you want?" She can then hand you the picture to make the request, with a gentle prompt if needed. If your child is not speaking yet and does not know how to communicate her wants and needs using pictures, you can teach her to use the Picture Exchange Communication program, commonly referred to as the PECS program. Contact information for the PECS program is listed in the Resources at the back of this book.
- If your child can speak a little, you can prompt by saying, "Say, 'I want . . . ,' " and then leave it to him to fill in the blank.

Even if you think you may know what your child wants, it's better to prompt him to request it than to give it to him right away. This is why we suggest you place objects that he likes or uses often in places where he can see them but not reach them. This way he'll have more opportunities to practice his requesting skills.

Here is another example: Suppose you're at the market and your child is sitting in the shopping cart. You walk down the cereal aisle, and as you reach for the box of his favorite cereal your child is smiling and becoming increasingly excited. As you grasp the box, he reaches for it but begins to frown when you don't offer him any. As you place it in the cart behind him, he watches your movement closely; he may reach for the box of cereal, but when he can't reach it, he begins to frown and fuss. If you continue down the aisle, he'll likely become very sad and cry. His initial reach for the box would have been the best moment to stop and prompt your child to request some of the cereal by pointing to it. But even if you missed the first opportunity, once you realize that he really wants it you can still prompt him to request it by pointing to it and looking at you. Then, of course, reinforce the pointing by giving him a few pieces. This is a good idea *even* at times when you don't really want him to have the cereal, like while you're still shopping in the store.

It's very important that your child learn to ask for the things he wants, even when he's upset. Later you can teach him how to wait for things or to understand a "*first* we do this/*then* we do that" kind of instruction (see the last section in this chapter). But until he understands those things, it's probably better to open the box of cereal and offer him a few pieces than to have him become upset and frustrated because he can't communicate his requests effectively. Think of it as a great opportunity to work on requesting when upset, which is such an important skill. *But* require him to point to the box or request it in an appropriate way, preferably followed by looking at you (you can help him do that by holding the box near your face and physically help him make a point if needed) before you give him the cereal; otherwise you'll just be reinforcing a tantrum!

Here is another example: Say you're in the park with your child and she's in a stroller. She sees another child feeding bits of bread to the ducks in a pond. She's very interested in the ducks and begins straining to get out of her stroller. Even though you know what she wants, and you could let her out of the stroller without having her ask to get out, you could use this as a learning opportunity. You could do this in several ways. You could prompt her to point to the ducks and then look at you. Or you could prompt her to use a gesture to communicate that she wants to be taken out of the stroller, by holding her arms up to you while making eye contact. Or you could offer her a picture of a duck, if you brought one, and direct her to hand it to you. What's nice about teaching these natural gestures and using pictures in these kinds of everyday situations is that the reinforcer is built in! Taking the child out of the stroller will be a natural and powerful reinforcer for her having requested it. After all, that is exactly what she wants most at that moment.

TEACHING YOUR CHILD TO COMMUNICATE WHEN HE *DOESN'T* WANT SOMETHING

Another skill that can help to prevent problem behavior is to teach children how to say "no" to the things they don't want and how to ask nicely for "help" or for "a break" or to be "all done" with an activity they wish to stop. If you think about problem behavior as a means of communicating for a child who has no other way to communicate, then it's important to give the child a way to say "No thank you"! Even if you really want your child to do something that he doesn't want to do, it's better for him to say "no" than to engage in problem behavior to communicate that message. It's important to remember that when you start trying to teach a child to use appropriate means of communicating "No thank you," you must always acknowledge the request and honor it as often as you can. Eventually, when your child is good at using words, gestures, signs, or handing you a picture to say "No thank you" or ask for a break, there will be time to teach him that he can't always have what he wants and can't always "opt out" when he wishes to do so. In the beginning, when he's learning to ask for a break or for help or to be all done, it's very important to reinforce every request, whenever possible, by giving him what he's asking for.

"All Done"

To teach this skill, think about situations your child tends to try to escape from or avoid. A common example is the dinner table; children often become bored and begin to whine and cry when they're finished eating and want to leave the table. This is especially true of young children in high chairs who cannot leave on their own; for children who also can't yet talk, this can be a particularly frustrating time. If this is the case with your child, you can teach her to point or use gestures, such as raising her arms to be picked up, to communicate that she wants to get out of her high chair.

Another idea is to place an "all done" picture on the table or tray in front of her that is well within her reach (you can copy the sign for "all done" shown below). As soon as you see that your child has finished eating and is beginning to squirm, prompt her to hand you the "all done" picture by helping her pick it up and hand it to you. Then say, "All done!" and help her down from the table immediately. Over time, fade your prompts until she's independently requesting to be all done by handing you the picture, signing "all done" or saying "all done." See the box on page 209 for more on using pictures to communicate requests.

If you prefer, you can also teach your child to make the sign for all done. One advantage to this method is that he will be able to use it any time, whether or not the pictures are available to him (on the other hand, the meaning of the pictures may be clearer to other adults). The sign for "all done" is shown below.

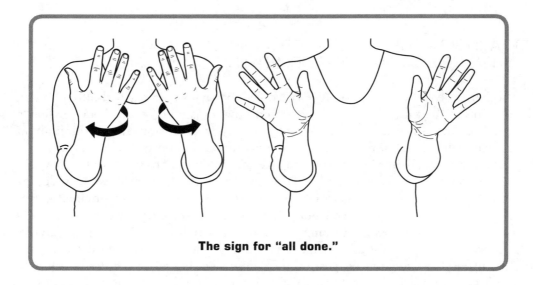

The sign for "all done."

CREATING PICTURES FOR YOUR CHILD TO MAKE REQUESTS

Teaching your child signs or other gestures to communicate important requests and responses like "yes," "no," and "all done" is very useful since these signs are portable. But you might find it helpful to start with pictures that represent these requests. You can use PECS as mentioned above (see the Resources). If you decide to try this, the important factor to keep in mind is that the pictures need to be simple and clearly differentiated from each other, preferably by color as well as symbol or shape. For example, you can create a "no" or "stop" picture on a sheet of paper by outlining your hand in a typical "stop" position (think of the way a crossing guard holds up a hand to stop traffic) and then coloring it in with red marker. Or you can color in a big bold "X" with a bright red crayon or marker. You can add the word "NO" in bold black letters inside the hand or under the "X" if you wish, but words aren't necessary (and your child doesn't need to be able to read them but just to recognize the picture with practice). Especially with very young children, it's important that the pictures look as different from one another as possible, so you could make a "yes" or "go" picture by coloring in a big check mark in a bright green.

To teach the child to use the pictures to communicate, prompt her to take the picture, preferably off a surface rather than from your hand, and then to hand the picture to you. Let's say you're feeding your child and the picture for "no" is on the tray of the high chair. You can ask, "More eggs?" and as soon as your child turns away or looks upset, use one of your hands to prompt her to pick up the picture of "no" and place it into your other hand. It's much better if there are two adults to do this at first—one to prompt from behind and the other to receive the picture and say, "Oh! No thank you! Okay, no more eggs," and then withdraw the spoon. In the beginning, the "prompt" may be hand-over-hand, whereas over time you can fade the prompt, just moving the child's arm toward the picture, and then phasing it out altogether.

In the beginning, the best way to teach this sign is to model it while saying, "All done," and then gently place your hands over your child's hands and help her make the sign for "all done" as you say "all done" again. Then immediately help her finish the activity (such as taking her out of her high chair) or removing a food, toy, or other item with which she wants to be finished. If you notice that she is beginning to try to make the sign by herself or to finish it once you've helped her start, you should begin to give her less and less help until eventually she can do it by herself. If she doesn't seem to begin or finish the gesture independently, after you've done this 50–100 times, try just placing your child's hands into position and see if she'll make the sign herself. If she does make the sign, or even an approximation of the sign, say, "You are all done," and immediately help her finish. If she does not make the sign herself, just continue to give her all the help she needs to successfully communicate that she is finished, delaying your help every now and then to see if she will begin to approximate the sign herself. Once she does, you should fade your prompting, giving her less and less help until she is doing it by herself. And, if you think the sign is too difficult for your child, it's fine to come up with your own sign and teach her that instead.

"No"

"No" is also a very important word or gesture to teach. After all, we're all entitled to say "No, thank you" when someone offers us a food we don't prefer or asks us to join in an activity we don't enjoy or aren't in the mood for. Be on the lookout for times that you offer your child something or ask him if he would like to do something and he suddenly runs, screams, or jerks his head away quickly. Wait until he's calm before offering it again, but this time immediately prompt him to shake his head no or put up his hand in a gesture that means "no" or to use the sign for "no," shown below. If this sign seems too difficult for his little hands to reproduce, try teaching the child just to shake his head no or use a picture as described in the box on page 209.

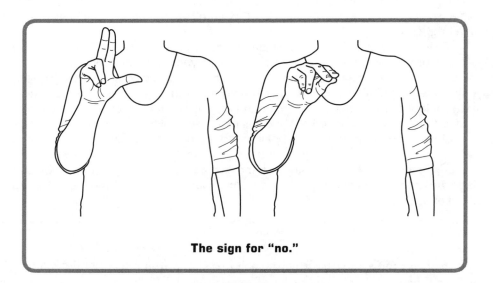

The sign for "no."

As soon as he begins making the prompted gesture, say, "No thank you!" and remove the offered item. A good place to practice this is during dinner. You can occasionally offer food choices that you know your child does not prefer, prompt him to make the gesture or hand you the picture for "No thank you!" and then remove the food you've offered.

"Help"

Finally, the word "help" is an important word or gesture to teach. The more your child can ask for help, by handing you a picture, the better. A common way to picture "help" is an outline of an upright hand with "HELP" written on it. Use a color that's different from that used for other pictures you're using and teach your child to use the picture as described in the box on page 209. Or teach your child to use a sign (shown below). Again, look for situations in which your child is struggling with something. You can also create situations in which your child will need your help. For example, put a favorite treat into a small, clear plastic container with a tight lid so that your child can see the treat but can't open the container to get it. As soon as you see him try to open the container unsuccessfully or show even the slightest frustration, prompt him to hand you the "help" picture or use a physical prompt to help him make the gesture that means "help" and then, as he is making the gesture or handing you the picture, say, "Help!" and then help him immediately.

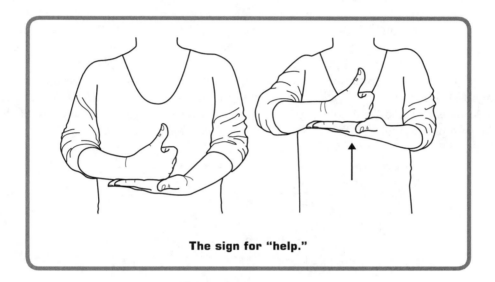

The sign for "help."

PROMPTING SPEAKING

We've been talking about how to teach nonverbal children (that is, children who can't talk) how to protest or communicate their desires for all done, break, no, help, something they want, and so forth, without crying, whining, or engaging in problem behavior. If your child *can* talk, or is good at imitating sounds and words, of course, you can and should use words to prompt your child to say "No" or "No thank you" if she can. You can also prompt her to say "All done" or "Break" or "I want a break" or "Help" or any of the words you would like her to learn to use when she is frustrated or upset.

The more practice you can give your child in making requests when he is *not* upset, the easier it will be for him to communicate requests, either with a point, a sign, a picture, or a word. And the easier it is for him, the more likely it is that he will be able to do it even when he's starting to get upset, which should help to prevent or reduce problem behavior.

FIRST . . . , THEN . . .

Another technique that may help your child tolerate some frustration is a "first . . . , then . . ." board. Showing the child two or three pictures of events that are going to happen in sequence can help her wait more patiently for a desired activity. This is especially important for children who have a lot of difficulty understanding spoken language.

Here's an example of how it might work: Say you're going to the bank and then the playground. Your child loves going to the playground and seems excited when you put some of his favorite playground toys into the car. To prevent him from becoming upset when you don't drive directly to the playground, it might help to do the following before you leave. First, show him two pictures, one of the bank and the other of the playground, stuck on a Velcro strip (see the drawing below). Label each picture as you point to it in turn, saying, "FIRST bank, THEN playground." Say this several times. Then let him hold the pictures (if he wants to) in the car. When you get to the bank, remind him, "FIRST bank, THEN playground." Make the bank trip short (practice this when you're getting cash, not negotiating a mortgage!). Then, as you get back in the car, point to the picture of the bank and say, "BANK is finished." Remove the bank picture and then point to the picture of the playground, saying, "NOW it's time for playground. Yay! Nice waiting!"

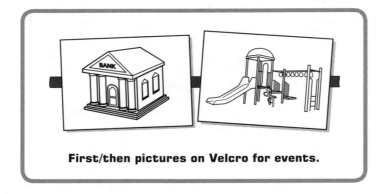

First/then pictures on Velcro for events.

We hope that using the techniques in this chapter for replacing problem behavior with simple communication will prevent or reduce problem behavior. If these techniques don't help, if you feel you need more guidance to implement them effectively, or if problem behavior seems more severe than in other children about the same age, please talk to your pediatrician about getting professional help.

Appendix

ACTIVITY LISTS

Y ou may find it helpful to reproduce these lists and keep them for handy reference in the areas where you perform each daily routine. The page numbers refer to where you'll find the instructions for each. Feel free to photocopy, or you can download and print them from *www.guilford.com/fein-forms*. Many parents find it helpful to wrap them in plastic or laminate them.

WAKING UP AND GOING TO SLEEP

Babies

Toddlers

DRESSING, UNDRESSING, AND DIAPER CHANGING

Babies

0–3 Months

Feels So Good! (page 134)
I Can Make It Happen! (page 134)
What Do I See? (page 134)
Tum-Tum on the Tummy (page 135)

3–6 Months

Baby Massage (page 148)
Go–Stop! (page 148)
What's Coming? (page 148)
Where's Mommy? (page 149)
Funny Mommy! (page 149)
Sock Off! (page 149)

6–9 Months

Peekaboo! (page 163)
Dressing Song (page 163)
Look at Mama! (page 163)
Yummy Baby! (page 164)

9–12 Months

Can I Have It? (page 179)
Which Socks? (page 179)
Shirt On, Shirt Off (page 179)
Where's Baby's Arm? (page 179)
Diaper Song (page 179)
Silly Mommy/Daddy! (page 180)

Toddlers:

1. Hello–Goodbye   LANGUAGE/PRETEND PLAY/IMITATION (page 66)
2. The Peekaboo Game   EYE CONTACT/SOCIAL ENGAGEMENT/THINKING (page 67)
3. Sticky, Wet, Open, Close   LANGUAGE (page 68)
4. The Diaper Song   LANGUAGE/SOCIAL ENGAGEMENT (page 69)
5. Red Shirt or Blue Shirt?   LANGUAGE/NONVERBAL COMMUNICATION (page 69)
6. Dressing Mr. Teddy   PRETEND/IMITATION (page 70)
7. Sock On, Sock Off!   SOCIAL ENGAGEMENT/LANGUAGE (page 70)
8. Where Did Baby Go?   SOCIAL ENGAGEMENT/LANGUAGE/THINKING (page 71)
9. Getting the Pants   LANGUAGE/THINKING (page 71)
10. Mommy's Shirt, Baby's Shirt   LANGUAGE/IMITATION/THINKING (page 72)
11. Silly Dressing   SOCIAL ENGAGEMENT/THINKING (page 73)

MEALTIME

Babies

3–6 Months

Kangaroo Cuddle (page 147)
You Do, I Do! (page 147)
How Many Tickles? (page 147)
Let's Touch! (page 148)

6–9 Months

Yummy/Yucky (page 162)
Here Comes the Plane (page 162)
Feed Mommy? (page 163)
Where Did It Go? (page 163)

9–12 months

Drinks for Everyone (page 177)
I Make Mommy/Daddy Honk! (page 177)
Fun with Food! Squish, Squish! (page 177)
Where Is It Hiding? (page 177)
Baby's First Words (page 178)
Let's Pretend! (page 178)
Which One Do We Want? (page 178)
I Can Feed Myself! (page 179)

Toddlers

1. More Cheese, Please   NONVERBAL COMMUNICATION/EYE CONTACT (page 74)

2. Grapes or Blueberries?   NONVERBAL COMMUNICATION (page 75)

3. Using Pictures to Request   NONVERBAL COMMUNICATION/EYE CONTACT (page 76)

4. Picture Menu   NONVERBAL COMMUNICATION (page 76)

5. Here Comes the Spoon!   EYE CONTACT (page 77)

6. Silly Mommy!   NONVERBAL COMMUNICATION/LANGUAGE (page 78)

7. Hot and Cold   LANGUAGE (page 79)

8. "Cut," "Big," and "Little"   LANGUAGE (page 79)

9. Counting with Food   LANGUAGE (page 80)

10. Teaching Color Words   LANGUAGE (page 81)

11. Verbal Imitation in the Kitchen   LANGUAGE/IMITATION (page 81)

12. Hide and Seek in the Rice   LANGUAGE/THINKING (page 81)

13. Fits or Doesn't Fit   LANGUAGE/THINKING (page 82)

14. Pretending to Feed Dolly   PRETEND PLAY/IMITATION (page 82)

15. Pretending to Cook   PRETEND PLAY/IMITATION/LANGUAGE (page 82)

16. Yummy/Yucky Food   LANGUAGE/THINKING (page 83)

17. Yummy and Yucky Toothpaste   LANGUAGE (page 84)

18. Getting Ready for Tooth Brushing   LANGUAGE/IMITATION (page 84)

19. Brushing Dolly's Teeth   IMITATION/PRETEND PLAY (page 84)

20. Fun with Food   BEHAVIOR, PRETEND, THINKING, IMITATION (page 85)

BATHTIME

Babies

0–3 Months

Just Right! (page 135)
Look at Me! (page 135)
What Do I See? (page 135)
What Do I Feel? (page 136)

3–6 Months

Let's Blow Bubbles (page 149)
Surprise Bags (page 149)
Bubble Bath (page 150)
Line 'Em Up and Knock 'Em Down
　(page 150)
Washcloth Games (page 150)

6–9 months

Rainbow Bathtime (page 164)
Drawing in the Tub (page 164)

6–9 months (continued)

Let's Go Fishing (page 164)
Fill and Spill (page 165)
Pop the Bubble (page 165)
Silly Ice Cubes (page 165)

9–12 Months

Mommy/Daddy Says (page 180)
Splash with Your Feet (page 180)
Ready, Set, Go! (page 180)
In and Out (page 181)
Dry and Wet (page 181)
Sticks/Doesn't Stick (page 181)
Body Parts (page 181)
Pretend (page 181)
Sink and Float (page 182)
Colors (page 182)

Toddlers

1. Wet and Dry, Head and Tummy　LANGUAGE (page 86)
2. I Splash, You Splash　IMITATION (page 87)
3. Bubbles on Body Parts　LANGUAGE (page 87)
4. Making Bathtub Choices　NONVERBAL COMMUNICATION (page 88)
5. Bath Songs　LANGUAGE (page 88)
6. Dolly's Bath　PRETEND PLAY/ LANGUAGE (page 89)
7. Splashing Hands and Feet　LANGUAGE (page 89)
8. Jump, Splash, Squirt　LANGUAGE (page 89)
9. Tub Toy Clean-Up　LANGUAGE/ NONVERBAL COMMUNICATION (page 90)
10. Sticks or Doesn't Stick　LANGUAGE/THINKING (page 90)
11. Floats or Sinks　LANGUAGE/THINKING (page 90)
12. Bathtub Colors　LANGUAGE/THINKING (page 91)
13. Fill and Spill　THINKING/LANGUAGE (page 91)
14. Drying Off Song　LANGUAGE/SOCIAL ENGAGEMENT (page 91)

CHORES

Babies

0–3 Months

Let's Wash the Clothes! (page 137)
I Smell Cinnamon! (page 137)

3–6 Months

Help Mommy Cook (page 151)
Funny Clean-Up (page 151)

6–9 Months

Laundry Time (page 166)
Baby Helping Mommy Cook (page 166)

9–12 Months

Laundry Time and Helping Mommy Cook
   (page 183)
Wash the Car (page 183)
Paint the House (page 183)
What Do I Hear? (page 184)

Toddlers

1. Driving to the Washing Machine   NONVERBAL COMMUNICATION/
   LANGUAGE/PRETEND PLAY (page 92)
2. The Laundry Routine   EYE CONTACT/NONVERBAL COMMUNICATION (page 93)
3. Laundry Language   LANGUAGE (page 94)
4. Laundry Matching   LANGUAGE/THINKING (page 94)
5. Where Does It Go?   THINKING (page 95)
6. The Clean-Up Song   THINKING/BEHAVIOR (page 96)
7. Clean-Up Sorting   THINKING (page 96)
8. Sorting Silverware   THINKING (page 97)
9. Washing the Table   IMITATION (page 97)
10. Sweep, Sweep, Sweep!   IMITATION (page 98)

ERRANDS

Babies

0–3 Months

We're Going in the Car! (page 136)
We're Going for a Walk! (page 136)
Let's Work Out! (page 136)

3–6 Months

We're Going for a Walk (page 151)
"Ba" and "Da" (page 151)
Help Mommy Shop (page 151)

6–9 Months

Baby Signs (page 165)

9–12 Months

Help Mommy/Daddy Shop (page 182)
Which One Do You Want? (page 182)
Word of the Day (page 183)

Toddlers

1. Waving Bye-Bye   NONVERBAL COMMUNICATION/EYE CONTACT/IMITATION (page 99)

2. Songs in the Car   LANGUAGE (page 100)

3. The Color Sighting Game   THINKING (page 100)

4. Pretend Car or Bus Trips   PRETEND PLAY (page 101)

5. Stop and Go   LANGUAGE (page 102)

6. Picture Schedule for Places We Go   THINKING/LANGUAGE (page 102)

7. The Errand Song   LANGUAGE/THINKING (page 103)

8. Remembering Pictures of Places   LANGUAGE/THINKING (page 104)

9. Waiting Patiently   BEHAVIOR/THINKING (page 104)

10. Stay with Me   BEHAVIOR (page 104)

11. From Market Matching to Visual Shopping Lists   THINKING/LANGUAGE/BEHAVIOR (page 105)

12. Where Does Baby Go?   LANGUAGE (page 106)

13. How Many Oranges?   LANGUAGE/THINKING/EYE CONTACT (page 106)

PLAYTIME

Babies

0–3 Months

Rhymes and Songs for Baby (page 137)
Really! You Don't Say! (page 138)
A Walk around the House (page 138)
Let's Move! (page 138)
Let's Look! (page 138)
Let's Touch! (page 139)
Let's Listen! (page 139)
Tummy Time (page 139)

3–6 Months

I Can Sit! (page 152)
I Can Reach and Roll (page 152)
Real-World Toys (page 152)
Peekaboo and Hide and Seek (page 152)
I Do, You Do! (page 153)
I Can Move Things (page 153)
Family Album (page 153)
Pinwheel (page 153)
Trot-Trot to Boston (page 154)
Bounce Time (page 154)
Way Up High (page 154)
Helium Balloon (page 154)
Disguise Face (page 155)
Songs for Moving Hands (page 155)

6–9 Months

Animal Tickles or Kisses (page 166)
Ahhhhhhhhh Boom! (page 166)
Vehicle Rides (page 166)
Now It's . . . (page 167)
Touch and Feel Box (page 167)
Paper Towel Roll Games (page 167)
Music Maker (page 167)
Play Ball! (page 168)
Let's Move (page 168)
Where's Baby? (page 169)
Pop-Up Time (page 169)
Find the Noise (page 169)
Where Is Thumbkin? (page 169)
Mirror Play (page 169)

9–12 Months

Let's Draw! (page 184)
Let's Talk! (page 184)
Baby Basketball (page 184)
Balloons (page 185)
Where's Your Nose? (page 185)
Nothing Can Go Wrongo (page 185)
Let's Unwrap (page 186)
Where's Mommy/Daddy? (page 186)
Sticks, Doesn't Stick (page 186)
Sand Table or Sandbox (page 186)
Stacking Rings, Blocks, Puzzles (page 187)
Tug of War (page 187)
Let's Swing (page 187)
Treasure Hunt (page 188)

PLAYTIME

Toddlers

Indoor Play

1. Color Matching and Color Words   LANGUAGE/THINKING (page 108)

2. Puzzle Piece Scavenger Hunt   LANGUAGE/THINKING/NONVERBAL COMMUNICATION (page 109)

3. Look Where I'm Looking!   NONVERBAL COMMUNICATION/SOCIAL ENGAGEMENT (page 110)

4. It's Still There!   LANGUAGE/THINKING (page 111)

5. Building Block Towers   LANGUAGE (page 111)

6. Playing with Balloons   LANGUAGE/MOTOR COORDINATION/EYE CONTACT (page 112)

7. Let's Play Ball!   NONVERBAL COMMUNICATION, EYE CONTACT, MOTOR COORDINATION, SOCIAL ENGAGEMENT (page 113)

8. Find the Music   THINKING (page 114)

9. Making Music   NONVERBAL COMMUNICATION, LANGUAGE (page 114)

10. Dance to the Music   EYE CONTACT, LANGUAGE, SOCIAL ENGAGEMENT (page 115)

11. The Singing Puppet   SOCIAL ENGAGEMENT (page 115)

12. Feed the Puppet   IMITATION/PRETEND PLAY (page 116)

13. Animal Time   LANGUAGE/PRETEND PLAY (page 116)

14. The Very Big Ball   LANGUAGE/EYE CONTACT/SOCIAL ENGAGEMENT (page 117)

15. I Want That One!   NONVERBAL COMMUNICATION/EYE CONTACT (page 117)

Outdoor Play

1. Let's Go Sliding!   LANGUAGE (page 118)

2. Sliding with Friends   SOCIAL ENGAGEMENT, BEHAVIOR (page 119)

3. Let's Go Swinging!   EYE CONTACT/NONVERBAL COMMUNICATION/LANGUAGE (page 119)

4. Drawing with Sidewalk Chalk   IMITATION/THINKING/MOTOR (page 121)

5. Bubbles, Bubbles, Bubbles!   EYE CONTACT/NONVERBAL COMMUNICATION/IMITATION/ MOTOR SKILLS (page 121)

6. Sand and Water   LANGUAGE/THINKING/EYE CONTACT/NONVERBAL COMMUNICATION (page 122)

7. Mixing Colors at the Water Table or the Sink   THINKING/NONVERBAL COMMUNICATION (page 123)

8. More Water Play   LANGUAGE/IMITATION (page 123)

9. Watering Can Sprinkling   LANGUAGE (page 123)

10. Scooter, Wagon, Tricycle, Toy Car   LANGUAGE/EYE CONTACT (page 124)

Resources

BOOKS TO READ TO YOUNG CHILDREN

Reading books to young children is a wonderful way to teach and reinforce early concepts as well as a terrific way to share and enjoy time together.

Leslie Patricelli has written a series of books that focus on a single concept and are great for teaching concepts to young children:

Yummy Yucky

Big Little

Happy Sad

No No Yes Yes

Quiet Loud

Higher Higher

Faster Faster

Huggy Kissy

Tickle

Potty

Tubby

Bill Martin, Jr., and Eric Carle (some written by Eric Carle alone) have a series of books with simple, recursive language:

Brown Bear, Brown Bear, What Do You See?

Polar Bear, Polar Bear, What Do You Hear?

Panda Bear, Panda Bear, What Do You See?

Does a Kangaroo Have a Mother Too?

The Very Hungry Caterpillar

Fiona Watts has written a lovely series of touch and feel books that emphasize adjectives:

That's Not My Dinosaur	*That's Not My Monkey*
That's Not My Puppy	*That's Not My Pig*
That's Not My Train	*That's Not My Lamb*
That's Not My Snowman	*That's Not My Truck*
That's Not My Teddy	*That's Not My Dragon*

Karen Katz has written a series of books that are great for teaching body parts, prepositions, and simple words:

Where Is Baby's Belly Button?	*I Can Share!*
Toes, Ears, and Nose	*A Potty for Me*
Excuse Me	*The Babies on the Bus*
What Does Baby Say?	*Baby Loves Winter*
What Does Baby Love?	*Baby Loves Spring*
How Does Baby Feel?	*Baby Loves Summer*
Where Is Baby's Mommy?	*Baby Loves Fall*
Baby's Colors	

DK Publishing publishes a series of lift-the-flap peekaboo books, which are great for teaching single words and the concept "Where is . . . ?":

Baby Faces Peekaboo	*Rainbow Colors Peekaboo*
Eyes, Nose, and Toes Peekaboo	*Bathtime Peekaboo*
Bedtime Peekaboo	*Playtime Peekaboo*
Farm Peekaboo	*Dress Up Peekaboo*

Sandra Boynton has a series of cheerfully written books that focus on early concepts such as emotions, clothing, counting, opposites, and letters:

Happy Hippo Angry Duck	*Are You a Cow?*
Blue Hat Green Hat	*Horns to Toes and in Between*
A to Z	*Bath Time*
Opposites	*Pajama Time*
One, Two, Three	*Tickle Time*

Additional classic early children's books mentioned in this volume:

Goodnight Moon by Margaret Wise Brown
Jesse Bear, What Will You Wear? by Nancy White Carlstrom

BOOKS TO INSPIRE PARENTS WITH IDEAS FOR TEACHING AND PLAY

The following books offer wonderful ideas for how to keep your child's attention during play and daily activities as well as offering many suggestions for early learning targets.

The Encyclopedia of Infant and Toddler Activities for Children Birth to 3 by Kathy Charner, Maureen Murphy, and Charlie Clark (Gryphon House, 2006).

The Toddler's Busy Book: 365 Creative Games and Activities to Keep Your 1½- to 3-Year-Old Busy by Trish Kuffner (Meadowbrook, 1999).

The Eentsy Weentsy Spider: Fingerplays and Action Rhymes by Joanna Cole and Stephanie Calmensonn (HarperCollins, 1991).

Funny Food: 365 Fun, Silly, Healthy Creative Breakfasts by Bill Wurtzel and Claire Wurtzel (Welcome Books, 2012).

Snacktivities: 50 Edible Activities for Parents and Young Children by MaryAnn F. Kohl (Gryphon House, 2001).

AUTISM-SPECIFIC TITLES

Behavioral Intervention for Young Children with Autism: A Manual for Parents and Professionals by Catherine Maurice (ProEd, 1996).

A Work in Progress: Behavior Management Strategies and a Curriculum for Intensive Behavioral Treatment of Autism by Ron Leaf and John McEachin (DRL Books, 1999).

An Early Start for Your Child with Autism: Using Everyday Activities to Help Kids Connect, Communicate, and Learn by Sally J. Rogers, Geraldine Dawson, and Laurie A. Vismara (Guilford Press, 2012).

101 Games and Activities for Children with Autism, Asperger's, and Sensory Processing Disorders by T. Delaney (McGraw-Hill, 2009).

Does My Child Have Autism? A Parent's Guide to Early Detection and Intervention in Autism Spectrum Disorders by Wendy L. Stone and Theresa Foy DiGeronimo (Jossey-Bass, 2006).

My Friend with Autism: A Coloring Book for Peers and Siblings by Beverly Bishop (Future Horizons, 2003).

Autism Solutions: How to Create a Healthy and Meaningful Life for Your Child by Ricki Robinson (Harlequin, 2011).

Reaching Out, Joining In: Teaching Social Skills to Young Children with Autism and Other Developmental Disabilities by Mary Jane Weiss and Sandra Harris (Woodbine House, 2001).

Siblings of Children with Autism: A Guide for Families by Sandra Harris and Beth Glasberg (Woodbine House, 3rd Edition, 2012).

Autism 24/7: A Family Guide to Learning at Home and in the Community by Andy Bondy and Lori Frost (Woodbine House, 2008).

FURTHER READING ON SPECIFIC TOPICS

When Children Don't Sleep Well: Interventions for Pediatric Sleep Disorders: Parent Workbook by Mark V. Durand (Oxford University Press, 2008).

Married with Special Needs Children: A Couple's Guide to Keeping Connected by Laura Marshak and Fran P. Prezant (Woodbine House, 2007).

Uncommon Father: Reflections on Raising a Child with a Disability by Donald J. Meyer (Woodbine House, 1995).

Toilet Training in Less Than a Day by Nathan Azrin and Richard Foxx (Pocket Books, 1989).

Toilet Training for Individuals with Autism or Other Developmental Disabilities by Maria Wheeler (Future Horizons, 2nd Edition, 2007).

Let's Talk Together—Home Activities for Early Speech and Language Development by Cory Poland and Amy Chouinard (Talking Child, 2008).

WEBSITES WITH PLAY IDEA LISTS FOR YOUNG CHILDREN

These websites list ideas for indoor and outdoor games and crafts to play with toddlers and preschoolers. Some list additional information on topics such as health and nutrition and/or offer general parenting tips.

Kids Fun and Games
www.kids-fun-and-games.com/index.html

Kid'sHealth
www.kidshealth.org/parent/growth/learning/toddler_games.html

BabyCenter
www.babycenter.com/preschooler-gamezties
www.babycenter.com/302_activities-play_1517839.bc

Family Education
www.familyeducation.com/home

www.ican.org.uk has excellent activity suggestions for parents.

Baby Signs
www.babysignlanguage.com has free information and videoclips of signs.

www.babysignstoo.com and *www.signbabies.com* have flash cards and other products for purchase.

PICTURE EXCHANGE COMMUNICATION SYSTEM

The Picture Exchange Communication System is a unique alternative/augmentative communication system for individuals with disabilities. There is a great deal of research supporting its efficacy in helping children with disabilities begin to initiate communication and in supporting the development of more complex forms of communication.

www.pecs.com

This website will familiarize you with the way PECS works, offer a variety of resources using PECS, from iPad apps to CD-ROMs with printable symbols, as well as information workshops and training near you.

The Picture Exchange Communication System Training Manual by Lori Frost and
   Andrew Bondy (Pyramid Educational Consultants, 2nd Edition, 2002).
PECS: *The Picture Exchange Communication System* by Lori Frost and Andrew
   Bondy (Pyramid Educational Consultants, 2nd Edition, 2002).

www.mayer-johnson.com/boardmaker-software

This website offers software that enables you to make icons for use with PECS.

WEBSITES FOR ORDERING EDUCATIONAL TOYS, TEACHING MATERIALS, ADAPTIVE MATERIALS, AND VISUAL TOOLS

Different Roads to Learning
www.difflearn.com

Lakeshore Learning
www.lakeshorelearning.com

Southpaw Enterprises
www.soutpawenterprises.com

Therapy Shoppe
www.therapyshoppe.com

Abilitations
www.abilitations.com

Special Needs Toys
www.specialneedstoys.com

Super Duper Publications
www.superduperpublications.com

National Autism Resources
www.nationalautismresources.com

Everyday Health
www.everydayhealth.com/autism/toys-and-games.aspx

Treezy
www.treezy.co.uk

Pro-Ed publisher
www.Proedinc.com

WEB RESOURCES

Help Me Grow
www.helpmegrownational.org

Help Me Grow is a system that connects at-risk children with the services they need.

Early Head Start
http://eclkc.ohs.acf.hhs.gov/hslc/tta-system/ehsnrc

Early Head Start provides early, continuous, intensive, and comprehensive child development and family support services to low-income infants and toddlers and their families and pregnant women and their families.

Easter Seals
www.easterseals.com

Easter Seals offers a huge range of information and services for children with disabilities. In particular, "Make the First Five Count" (*www.easterseals.com/mtffc*) is a program that raises awareness for children at risk for a variety of disabilities. Here you can find resources such as The Ages and Stages Questionnaire, a free online screening tool for parents to track their child's developmental milestones.

Parent to Parent USA
www.p2pusa.org

This organization matches each parent looking for information and support with an experienced parent of a child with special needs.

Sibling Support Project
www.siblingsupport.org

This website offers information about workshops, conferences, publications, and other opportunities for siblings of children with disabilities to become educated and connect with one another.

Child Law Center
www.childcarelaw.org/pubs-audience.shtml#parents

This website provides parent resources for child care for children with disabilities as well as information about the Americans with Disabilities Act and other laws affecting children with special needs.

Zero to Three
www.zerotothree.org/about-us/areas-of-expertise/free-parent-brochures-and-guides

This website includes many parenting resources, including a comprehensive list of early developmental milestones and ideas for supporting and optimizing your child's early development.

AUTISM-SPECIFIC WEB RESOURCES

Autism Speaks
www.autismspeaks.org

This website is one of the most comprehensive resources for families, including state-by-state information on local resources and services, and offers a 100-day kit to help families navigate the first 100 days after diagnosis, as well as providing news on current autism research and advocacy and toolkits for parents of newly diagnosed children.

Autism Society
www.autism-society.org

This website will lead individuals to the autism society in their particular state, which will have information on local resources, treatment providers, and events and often hosts a web support group for parents.

Families for Effective Autism Treatment
www.feat.org

This website will link individuals to the Families for Effective Autism Treatment organization in their state, which will have information on local resources, treatment providers, and events and in-person and online support groups for parents and other ways for parents to connect and share resources.

Children's Disabilities Information
www.childrensdisabilities.info/autism/index.html

This website lists support groups for parents of children with ASD.

Autism Science Foundation
www.autismsciencefoundation.org

ASF funds autism research and also provides useful information for parents on autism and evidence-based treatment options.

Rethink
www.rethinkfirst.com

This website provides Web-based teaching tutorials on ABA (applied behavior analysis), video images of teaching interactions, and teaching objectives, available for a monthly subscription.

Most states in the United States have a variety of services for parents of children at risk. These might include early intervention services for children with delayed development and family support services such as Family Resource Centers or the Nurturing Families Network. Check with your state Early Childhood or Early Intervention Office for information on the resources available in your state.

Behavior Analyst Certification Board has a list of board-certified behavior analysts in your area, by ZIP code.

INTERNATIONAL RESOURCES

International List of Organizations
www.autismspeaks.org/what-autism/world-autism-awareness-day/international-autism-organizations

Australia

www.seanasmith.com/books/the-australian-autism-handbook/

A comprehensive guide for parents navigating the early months after their child has been diagnosed with autism, with focus on services in Australia.

www.latrobe.edu.au/otarc/your-questions-answered

Provides answers to frequently asked questions and links to autism-related services and organizations in Australia.

www.autismaspergeract.com.au

Provides information and practical support to people involved in the autism community, including parent support groups and links to Australian organizations and services.

www.dss.gov.au/sites/default/files/documents/08_2014/6006_-_accessible_-_early_intervention_practice_guidelines_0.pdf

Provides information on early intervention for children with autism spectrum disorder by very well-known Australian autism researchers.

www.autismhelp.info

An initiative of Gateways Support Services. The website aims to increase awareness of autism spectrum disorder through providing practical strategies, information and resources to parents, teachers, child care workers and professionals, and provides information about some funds available for early intervention.

Canada

Autism Society of Canada
http://autismsocietycanada.ca

Provides information on autism and referrals to many helpful services and resources. ASC puts special focus on providing information, referral, and resources for parents and other family members who are seeking support for children with autism.

Autism Ontario
www.autismontario.com

A good source of information and referral on autism and a voice representing the autism community in Ontario. Links to information on ABA providers.

Canadian Autism Spectrum Disorders Alliance
www.asdalliance.org/English/index.html

CASDA is a national coalition of autism related professionals, family members, and community members working to secure the federal government's commitment to the development of a National Autism Action Plan.

Geneva Centre
www.autism.net/index.php

A service provider for the Toronto area.

Autism Speaks Canada
www.autismspeaks.ca

The Canada branch of Autism Speaks, with links to Canadian resources and events, and general information about autism.

United Kingdom

National Autistic Society
www.autism.org.uk

A long-established organization for autism advocacy. The website provides links to local services.

National Health Service
www.nhs.uk/Conditions/Autistic-spectrum-disorder

Provides links to information on health, support, and the benefits you are entitled to.

Simple Steps Autism
www.simplestepsautism.com

An online teaching platform for learning more about ABA—for purchase.

Skybound Therapies
www.skyboundtherapies.co.uk

A therapy center in West Wales for children with autism and a variety of other developmental disabilities. They serve local children but also provide consultants for developing home programs.

Treezy
www.treezy.co.uk

Educational and autism resources sold in the United Kingdom (the U.K. version of Different Roads to Learning).

Peach for Children with Autism
www.peach.org.uk

Links families with ABA providers across the United Kingdom.

Ireland (see also U.K. links)

Irish Autism Action
www.autismireland.ie

Advocacy organization that also provides links to service providers and a brief, clear description of major types of autism intervention.

Centre for Behavior Analysis, School of Education, Queens University, Belfast
www.qub.ac.uk/cba

Provides video links and short courses on topics within behavior analysis.

Index

f following a page number indicates a figure, t following a page number indicates a table.

DATE DUE

Deborah Fein, I————————————————fessor in the
Departments of————————————————of Connecticut.

Molly Helt, PhI————————————————of Psychology
and Neuroscien————————————————ild with autism.

Lynn Brennan, l————————————————analyst,
based in Massac————————————————autism
spectrum disorders for more than 20 years.

Marianne Barton, PhD, is Clinical Professor and Director of Clinical
Training in the Department of Psychology at the University of Connecticut,
where she is also Director of the Psychological Services Clinic.